Sou
Voices

Josephine Ensign

With a Foreword by Arthur W. Frank

Perspectives in Medical Humanities

Perspectives in Medical Humanities publishes peer reviewed scholarship produced or reviewed under the auspices of the University of California Medical Humanities Consortium, a multi-campus collaborative of faculty, students, and trainees in the humanities, medicine, and health sciences. Our series invites scholars from the humanities and health care professions to share narratives and analysis on health, healing, and the contexts of our beliefs and practices that impact biomedical inquiry.

General Editor

Brian Dolan, PhD, Professor of Social Medicine and Medical Humanities, University of California, San Francisco (UCSF)

Other Titles in this Series

Patient Poets: Illness from Inside Out
Marilyn Chandler McEntyre (Fall 2012) (Pedagogy in Medical Humanities series)

Bioethics and Medical Issues in Literature
Mahala Yates Stripling (Fall 2013) (Pedagogy in Medical Humanities series)

From Bench to Bedside, to Track & Field: The Context of Enhancement and its Ethical Relevance
Silvia Camporesi (Fall 2014)

Heart Murmurs: What Patients Teach Their Doctors
Edited by Sharon Dobie, MD (Fall 2014)

Follow the Money: Funding Research in a Large Academic Health Center
Henry R. Bourne and Eric B. Vermillion (Spring 2016)

www.UCMedicalHumanitiesPress.com

This series is made possible by the generous support of the Dean of the School of Medicine at UCSF, the Center for Humanities and Health Sciences at UCSF, and a Multicampus Research Program Grant from the University of California Office of the President. Grant ID MR-15-328363.

mh

Soul Stories
Voices from the Margins

Josephine Ensign

With a Foreword by Arthur W. Frank

First published in 2018
by University of California Medical Humanities Press

© 2018 by Josephine Ensign
University of California
Medical Humanities Consortium
3333 California Street, Suite 485
San Francisco, CA 94143-0850

Cover image used with permission © Josephine Ensign
Photos on pages 39 and 67 by Josephine Ensign.

Book design by Virtuoso Press.

Library of Congress Control Number: 2018944750
ISBN: 978-0-9963242-6-7

Printed in USA

To my children, Jonathan and Margaret

What kind of beast would turn its life into words?
What atonement is this all about?
—and yet, writing words like these, I am also living.
—Adrienne Rich

Contents

Foreword

Inviting the Other

The Buddhist teacher Pema Chödrön offers the blessing: "May we go to places that scare us." That may express best why I value the writing of Josephine Ensign. She takes us to places that, if they don't exactly frighten us, do unsettle us; places that disturb our comfort, that make us realize that we have become more complacent than we thought we ever would.

In the movements known variously as health humanities and narrative medicine, nurses have not been as vocal as their numbers would warrant. It may be indicative that Ensign's ongoing clinical nursing work is not in hospitals, but rather in what might best be called outreach clinics, because they serve those who would otherwise drift out of reach, those who need to be pulled back to some form of safety. In contemporary nursing, it may be most possible to speak from the margins. Ensign works in places where institutional strictures are looser because people's needs are more primary: something to eat, a place to sleep, a moment of feeling clean. In one of this book's most important chapters, nurses learn to wash the feet of people who are not, strictly, their patients. Calling them guests seems more appropriate. Ensign practices medicine in its most basic form of *hospitality*. She invites those who would not be welcome elsewhere, even in hospital emergency departments. Her clinical practice begins with making these people feel valued.

Ensign also can be funny. Maybe you have to have written some grant proposals to get the humor, and also the serious truth, of her career-changing decision to write based on her own experiences—personal, teaching, and clinical—rather than spending her time seeking funding to gather data. The data, she realizes, are already all around her. What's difficult is not gathering data; that requires fairly blunt effort. What's truly difficult is saying something about those data that moves people to do something differently, whether that doing differently takes place in readers' thoughts, their personal lives, their political lives as citizens, or their professional lives. Responding to this difficulty, this book is, on one level, a series of stylistic experiments in which Ensign plays with different ways of telling stories. Some of these experiments seem more successful than others, but I would not presume that all readers would agree with me as to which succeed best. Not least among the others whom Ensign invites to participate are her readers, to whom she grants more interpretive space than most academic arguments allow. Her stories' gaps call up one of the four types of interpretive questions that she proposes as important for readers to ask: about what is a story *silent*? In many of Ensign's silences, I hear her to be leaving an opening for readers to fill.

Three recurring currents of thought give unity to these experiments in narration. The first is Ensign's autobiographical turnings and returnings. When she encounters otherness—most often in conditions of homelessness—Ensign's first response is to ask herself when she has been where this other person now is. Her earlier book *Catching Homelessness* is more explicitly autobiographical, but readers who come directly to *Soul Stories* are told enough to fill in the background. Ensign's point is never to write about them, whether these others are the patients, the research subjects, the students, or other objects of the author's knowing gaze. Ensign does gaze at others, sometimes quite critically, but then she always sees herself, both herself having been where those others now are, and herself doing the gazing for motives that are always questionable. Here autobiography morphs into the second unifying current, self-reflection.

Just when Ensign's observations of a "coolly detached young woman physician" at a workshop veer toward bitterness at the overt display of privilege, Ensign stops to ask what demons this young woman might be trying to face, presenting herself as she does. When Ensign sits in a shoe store observing the buyers of fashionable footwear, she asks what her own boots say about herself. "Wearing the mantle of self-righteousness as if it were a hair shirt is something I have learned to be aware of and to shrug off before it sticks to me" (14). It's hard, very hard, to be a social critic, to try and tell truths about what is objectionably wrong, without lapsing into self-righteousness; some times the shirt is going to stick. But Ensign consistently turns her critical gaze back onto herself. Volunteering in a juvenile detention center, teaching young people to write, she reflects on how her work participates in a larger disciplinary apparatus: "*This* is how a love letter should be; *this* is how a poem should be: we altered their words, their sentences, their metaphors, trying to make them fit our notion of cathartic poetry. We five white adults who would walk out of juvie at the end of the day, see trees, see our families, sleep in our own beds" (17). I read that reflection as a comment on hospital work, as carried out by people who, hard working as they are, will go home to sleep in their own beds.

The third and most unifying current running through Ensign's experiments in narration is what I would call her politics of moral imagination. In these writings, her political concerns are not with organizing local responses to specific issues, though she works that territory, too. Here, her concern seems to be offering her readers a way of seeing the relations between privilege and radical need without our usual resistances. We resist recognizing privilege for what it is because that would require questioning our own privilege. And we resist recognizing others' need because that would obligate us to respond more expansively than we usually choose to.

Although Ensign begins the book by setting up a distance between her work and the program in narrative medicine at Columbia University, I read her as advancing the program called for most explicitly by the Columbia physician Sayantani DasGupta, whom she quotes. Something else DasGupta writes describes what Ensign is doing: "This work must be done with attention to power and privilege that attends to not simply the texts we read together, but the relational texts we live, breathe, and create in our classrooms and our workshop spaces." Ensign has, to my knowledge, gone further than anyone in asking how these "relational texts" are lived and created in community clinics, in health professional classrooms, in designated memorial sites, and in everyday settings like shoe stores. She reads these settings for how they sometimes question relations of power and privilege, but more often how they reinforce the status quo of who seems entitled to what. She makes the margins of the world her text, but it's a text that is constantly being rewritten by actions, including her writing and her readers' responses.

Throughout this book Josephine Ensign makes me look: she makes me look at others for whom I don't want to feel responsibility; she makes me look at who I choose to serve and associate with, and what I effect by those choices; and she makes me look at my own life, especially my systematic inattentions. Reading her, I realize that I have done my best work when I have felt the most immediate fellowship with those whom I wrote about; those blessed moments when witnessing the other is equally to witness one's own struggles, scars, and occasional triumphs.

To be generous, a person has to give up perfection. I can imagine a more perfectly edited version of this book. But difficult as it is for someone invested in an academic life to admit, that more perfect book might not be a better book. It would risk turning readers into passive admirers of the author's performance. Josephine Ensign does not want our admiration. She wants to see, to recognize, to feel, and to find ways to respond.

Arthur W. Frank

University of Calgary, Canada and VID Specialized University, Norway

Preface

One midwinter's day in Seattle in 2009, I sat at my desk at home writing a federal grant proposal for investigating ways to improve health care for homeless young people. I stopped typing midsentence and gazed out the window at the rain and wind rippling the bamboo leaves in my garden. I asked myself what I was doing with my life.

I was a tenured professor teaching community health and health policy to nursing students at a large university. I was a nurse practitioner working with homeless teens and young adults in a community clinic. I loved teaching and I loved my work as a nurse, but this type of writing was not what I longed to do. I needed to find a way to merge my work in health care with my love of writing—of real writing, not the stiff, academic, formulaic writing required by my academic job, and certainly not the cold, distant medical writing in my patient clinical chart notes. Real writing to me was expressive, creative writing—reflective writing that allowed the "I" back into the frame, as, of course, I am doing now. So, as if it were a crystal ball, I typed into my computer's search engine the words "healthcare" and "literature." Among the results were links to narrative medicine and to the Narrative Medicine program at Columbia University in New York City.

Developed over the past several decades by physician and literary scholar Rita Charon and her colleagues, narrative medicine (as defined by Charon) "fortifies clinical practice with the narrative competence to recognize, absorb, metabolize, interpret, and be moved by the stories of illness." Charon has developed a narrative medicine close reading drill that she teaches to health care students and professionals to help them achieve narrative competence. The close reading drill consists of paying attention to the following elements of a text or a patient story: (1) frame, such as "Where does this text come from? How did it appear? What does it answer? How was it answered?"; (2) form, including genre, visible structure, narrator, metaphor, allusion to other texts, and diction; (3) the use of time; (4) plot, or what happens in the story; and (5) desire, with desire being the answer to the question "What appetite is satisfied by virtue of the reading act?" Charon contends that having a cadre of narratively competent physicians, nurses, and other health care professionals contributes to improvements in the quality of health care, especially the provision of what has come to be called patient-centered care.

Patient-centered care, as defined by the Institute of Medicine in its 2001 *Crossing the Quality Chasm* report, is "providing care that is respectful of and responsive to individual patient preferences, needs, and values, and ensuring that patient values guide all clinical decisions." Charon concedes that the application of narrative medicine can add to the time required for a health care provider to ask for and listen to (and then hopefully do something to incorporate and act on) a patient's story of illness.

To aid in efficient patient-centered care, Charon and her narrative medicine colleague, the physician Sayantani DasGupta, advocate for patients to become narratively competent, to learn how to effectively organize their illness stories. DasGupta, as quoted in an *O, The Oprah Magazine* article, advises people to "choose the turning points you want to highlight—the ups and downs you've experienced over time. ... Mention the dramatic tensions. ... Finally, spill your fears." In this same article, Charon states that she begins a medical appointment with a new patient by stating, "Please share with me what I need to know," and then sits back and lets the patient tell her story.

Narrative medicine was intriguing as well as sufficiently academically rigorous for me to legitimately pursue as a topic within my academic position. I set out on a course of self-study, reading various books and academic journal articles on the topic. I attended the introductory and then the advanced workshop in narrative medicine at Columbia University, both led by Dr. Charon—one of these workshops I describe in this book's opening essay, "Soul Story." I then began to offer a series of weekly narrative medicine sessions at the university health sciences library at the university where I work. I called this series Poetry and Prose Rounds, and invited health care providers, students, patients, and family members of patients to read and discuss short pieces of poetry and prose. I then asked participants to respond to reflective writing prompts that were linked to themes discussed that day.

While I was attracted to the concept and stated purpose of narrative medicine, and it certainly did merge my love of literature with medicine, I began to question aspects of it.

I realized that narrative medicine discourse assumes an ideal encounter between an empathic physician and a resource-rich, cognitively intact, and compliant adult patient. I wondered: What does this mean for providers or patients who fall outside these parameters? What does it mean for people excluded from health care? What does it mean to be attuned not only to the narratives of individual patients or communities, but also to the larger, often silenced metanarratives of power and exclusion? By *metanarrative* I refer to the *Oxford English Dictionary* definition of "an archetypal story, which provides a schematic world view upon which an individual's experiences and perceptions may be ordered."

In its earlier form, narrative medicine allowed little room for reflexivity or exploration of the larger structural inequities and structural violence within health care, including those deriving from the medical gaze. *Medical gaze* is the term coined by French philosopher Michel Foucault to refer to the distancing, objectifying stance modern medicine takes towards diagnosing and treating human disease. Until more recently, narrative medicine largely ignored the limits of narrative, especially within the context of trauma, suffering, and oppression.

As both a health care provider and a teacher of health science students, I began to have concerns about the praxis of narrative medicine—where the rubber of theory hits the road of the practice of medicine, nursing, and health care. In this age of the quantified clinician, checklist manifestos, and medical simulation labs, presenting something as complex as literary critical theory in a drill format somehow misses the mark of what medical humanities can and should do well: opening up what the Irish physician Seamus O'Mahony calls "hinterland and perspective." O'Mahony defines *hinterland* as the connection with the broader culture beyond the narrow culture of biomedicine, and perspective as understanding modern medicine's place in society and in history. To O'Mahony's critique of narrative medicine, I add a more critical feminist and public health slant in order to foreground power, oppression, and social justice issues.

It should be noted that narrative medicine as a disciplinary field has matured and many of its leading practitioners have incorporated their own versions of similar critiques to those I describe above. For instance, Sayantani DasGupta writes eloquently about her awareness of the role of power and privilege inherent in both the provider-patient and teacher-student relationships that are at the core of narrative medicine. She calls for attention to these issues, stating, "Otherwise, even narrative work within healthcare risks carrying within its practices and pedagogies the potential to replicate the selfsame hierarchical, oppressive power dynamics of traditional medicine that the field is designed to address. Hence, narrative medicine must insist on a hypervigilance against exploitation of the inherent power of professional status."

An additional aspect of narrative medicine that continues to cause me discomfort is its highbrow and elitist stance, perhaps a side effect of its roots within the private Ivy League New York City institution of Columbia University—what with its own roots as King's College established in the mid-eighteenth century by charter of King George II—and of Rita Charon's doctorate in literature focusing on the work of Henry James. Heady and refined and intellectual and very Eurocentric. And so very not the irreverent West Coast me, and not most of the nursing students or patients or communities with whom I work.

I am a nurse providing health care to people marginalized by poverty and homelessness. I teach at a large public university in the still-frontier town of Seattle. Many of my students are first-generation immigrants and refugees from war-torn countries, or are from Washington State's rural farming or fishing families, the first to attend college. I am not a recent immigrant, nor a refugee, nor the first person in my family to attend college. But I am the product of resource-poor, racist, rural Southern public schools, and I did not have an easy childhood: poetry and books saved my life quite literally. As British writer Jeanette Winterson points out in her memoir, *Why Be Happy When You Could Be Normal?*, I recognize that literature is not something solely for the educated elite:

> So when people say that poetry is a luxury, or an option, or for the educated middle classes, or that it shouldn't be read at school because it is irrelevant, or any of the strange and stupid things that are said about poetry and its place in our lives, I suspect that the people doing the saying have had things pretty easy. A tough life needs a tough language—and that is what poetry is. That is what literature offers—a language powerful enough to say how it is. It isn't a hiding place. It is a finding place.

Literature has been my finding place, and so I have sought ways to share that potential within my work. Over the years, through my teaching and practice of narrative medicine in the classroom and in my health care encounters (as patient, as provider, and as family member of my elderly and dying parents), I developed and applied a more feminist, critical, emancipatory, and widely accessible close reading drill that I refer to as "the closer close reading drill." It includes the following four items, which I invite you to apply as you read *Soul Stories*:

- <u>Emotion</u>. What do you feel while reading this piece or while listening to this person's illness narrative? Where in your body do you most feel this emotion? What is the overall mood or emotional effect of the piece? And why do you think it evokes this particular response in you?

- <u>Surprise</u>. What stands out to you the most? What is unexpected? The word *surprise*, used here, is similar to Roland Barthes's term *punctum* in his book *Camera Lucida*, or is, as medical sociologist Arthur W. Frank states, "what distracts you but is not the focus of the narrative."

- <u>Silence</u>. What is unsaid in this piece? Whose voice or perspective is included and whose is left out, and why?

- <u>Metaphor and simile</u>. What are the instances of the use of imagery and the poetics of the piece? How are they used, and why?

And as for real writing within my own life? In retrospect, it was fortuitous that I submitted my last federal health care grant back in 2009, at a time of extreme funding cutbacks during our country's Great Recession. The reviewers' feedback was that it was a worthwhile proposal and that it would have received funding if it had come in a year or so earlier, when they had more money. Around that same time, I sat in a faculty meeting where a successful older researcher showed a PowerPoint slide with a series of rolling hills leading off into the distance and a road with National Institutes of Health (NIH) grant signs, one after the other, leading over the hills and fading into the sunset. Her point was that this was how our lives as university researchers should look: this slide represented our marching orders. I stared at the slide and then whispered to a colleague, "and then you die."

I have nothing against NIH or the researchers who stake their careers on NIH or similar grants, but I knew that slide did not represent the life I wanted. I was forty-nine years old at that point, and my mother had died the year before; the sunset in the slide seemed very real. My husband had also recently commented that if I had used the same amount of time, effort, ink, and paper that went into my grant-writing, I would have written a book manuscript—or several—by then.

Instead of revising and resubmitting my rejected NIH grant proposal, I began to write what became my first published book, a medical memoir titled *Catching Homelessness: A Nurse's Story of Falling Through the Safety Net*. This was a book about my work with and spiral into homelessness as a young adult. Through the writing of *Catching Homelessness*, I did what I consider real writing. The act of researching and writing the book, a book which wove in pertinent events from my personal as well as professional lives, helped give some narrative cohesion to my own fractured and oftentimes confusing existence.

While writing a later chapter of that book, "Greyhound Therapy," which deals with gender-based violence, I brushed up against a then mostly closed door to my own childhood traumas. I made the decision to keep that door closed: to open it within *Catching Homelessness* would have led away from the main purpose of the book, which was to illustrate the complexities involved with homelessness and its attendant ills. I knew that to open the new door would require a much different book, one that contextualized the effects of trauma on individuals and communities, and the ways that narrative and storytelling factor into health and healing.

That much different book became *Soul Stories: Voices from the Margins*. The opening of that door and the personal exploration of what was behind that door led to this book. In writing it, I allowed myself to stray from the clear objective facts of science and medicine into the murkier subjective part of what it means to be human, and what it means to find healing in the face of trauma. This book is the result of that labyrinthine journey.

Throughout *Soul Stories*, whenever I write about interactions with patients, I have changed certain biographical details and names in order to protect identities. I have not changed names or other identifying details of friends, co-workers, or family members, except where indicated as such within the text. In writing this book, I sought to speak the truth of my own story—even when that involved speaking truth to and against powerful entities—while attempting to steer clear of any score-settling vindictiveness or sensationalized tabloid tell-all. The questions I continuously asked myself while writing this book were these: Is this detail necessary for the telling of this story? Is this personal story necessary to illustrate the larger societal story I am attempting to tell?

Soul Stories is an exploration of the boundaries of narrative within health and healing, in the context of trauma and homelessness. It draws on scholarly research across a range of disciplines, and is informed by my thirty years' experience as a nurse providing health care to people marginalized by poverty and homelessness, by my personal journey through homelessness as a young adult, and by my experience teaching critical reflective practice to health science students. *Soul Stories* deepens our understanding of homelessness; trauma and resilience; gender-based violence; the role of narrative in health and healing; and ways in which we can humanize health care for patients, providers, and communities. It contributes to civically and community-engaged scholarship in the health humanities.

Health humanities is the relatively new field of inquiry linking health and social care disciplines with the arts and humanities. As stated by the International Health Humanities Network, of which I am an active member, health humanities "aims to encourage innovation and novel cross-disciplinary explorations of how the arts and humanities can inform and transform healthcare, health and well-being." Health humanities breaks out of the limited application of medical humanities—which focuses on the training of physicians—and includes work by informal and family caregivers, patients, and community groups.

With that wider audience in mind, my aim is for *Soul Stories* to be informed by research and academic writings, yet accessible to the general reader. *Soul Stories* expands narrative medicine through an exploration of the effects of trauma on individuals and communities, the complicated role of the witness, the limits of narrative and of narrative medicine, and ways for marginalized voices to be heard within health care.

One

Soul Story

I love all waste
And solitary places; where we taste
The pleasure of believing what we see
Is boundless, as we wish our souls to be.
—Percy Bysshe Shelley

One Sunday in early June 2012, the sole of my right foot split in two, weeping amber juices like an overripe nectarine. The split occurred while I was standing in the New York Public Library on Fifth Avenue, leaning over a display case and reading passages from Mary Wollstonecraft Shelley's "Journal of Sorrow." Her once private leather-bound journal was open, revealing pages of sepia-colored handwriting. Beside the journal lay a gold locket and a charred fragment of Percy Bysshe Shelley's skull. Information plaques explained that Percy drowned at age twenty-nine in a sailing accident off the coast of Italy, where he was living in exile with his wife, Mary, and their son. Percy's body washed up on shore a few days after the accident, reportedly with a copy of Sophocles's *Tragedies* in his coat pocket. He was cremated on the beach, but a friend saved fragments of his skull, as well as locks of his hair, which were later turned into a mourning locket.

It was late afternoon and I was taking a break from walking the length of Manhattan. I'd started in Lower Manhattan at the filled-in crater of the former Twin Towers, then walked north through a children's street fair in

Washington Park and up Fifth Avenue towards my monk's cell at Union Theological Seminary in Morningside Heights. I wore a pair of black rubber flip-flops, not good walking equipment for my long afternoon trek.

I savored being alone, not lonely, on the bustling streets of Manhattan, swept along in the river of people. A furious thunderstorm erupted when I passed the Empire State Building. As the first hard, scattered raindrops fell on the sidewalk, their steam redolent of rusty iron, I realized I had no umbrella. So, I hurried past the stone lions, up the external marble stairs, and ducked inside the library, where there was an exhibit, *Shelley's Ghost*.

The exhibit was in a small, dimly lit room on the main floor of the library. There were only a few people inside, along with a silent guard standing by the door. The room had the hushed, reverential air of cathedrals. I walked around the exhibit several times, drawn back to Mary's journal. Although it felt unseemly to read parts of her private grief, to peer into the written wound splayed open, I stood beside it mesmerized.

Thunder rumbling through the cavernous library, accompanied by a searing pain in my right foot, startled me out of my reverie. I felt as if I had been struck by lightning or seared by the hot coal of hell. Surrounded by Frankenstein, Gothic relics, and hair jewelry, anything was possible. I gasped from the pain, causing the guard to glower at me. Discreetly, I glanced down at my foot and saw that my sole had a gaping hole diagonally through the instep. In Western medical parlance, I had a ruptured subepidermal friction bullae, or a partial-thickness blister; in Eastern medical parlance I had a wounded solar plexus chakra. Whatever it was called, it hurt. Suddenly, being alone in the middle of Manhattan felt lonely.

I considered taking a taxi back to my room at the seminary where I was staying, but decided I could tough it out, walk back, and save money. After the storm had passed, I limped outside, then through puddles of floating refuse, gulley-washed into crosswalks, and past homeless people pushing compact shopping carts piled with tattered garbage bags stuffed with possessions. The recent hard rain intensified the miasma emanating from the pavement and from the crush of damp, soured bodies. I wondered what assortment of exotic germs of diseases from around the world, what sloughed-off skin cells from people, rats, pigeons, and poodles, I was absorbing through my open wound.

To distract myself from the pain and futile germ phobia, I pondered questions that had been flashing through my head like an existential version of the Nasdaq sign in Times Square: Why am I attracted to the suffering of others? What draws me to the pain, to the flowing juices of the wounded body? Why have I spent the past thirty years working as a nurse with homeless and marginalized people? Would I be happier—and able to afford a better pair of shoes—if I had been drawn to work as a shoe buyer for Saks Fifth Avenue? The latter question occurred to me as I hobbled past the wrought-iron-festooned display windows of Saks's flagship store.

I was in New York for a week to attend the narrative medicine advanced workshop at Columbia University's College of Physicians and Surgeons. The workshop consisted of thirty participants. Most were physicians, a few were nurses, and the rest were medical ethicists, hospital chaplains, and patient advocates. All were smart, intense, overachieving types. We were there to learn about ways to incorporate the stories of health, healing, and the human condition into our work. Our final session had been that morning, so I was now free to explore Manhattan and to reflect on what I had learned.

As I limped north along Fifth Avenue, I thought about how I am defined as much by my revulsions as by my attractions. In one of our last workshop sessions, we read and discussed Colm Toíbín's short story "One Minus One," a haunting story of family love, belonging, and regret. In the opening of the short story, the male protagonist is gazing at the full moon in Texas, which takes him back to the last real thing that happened to him: the death of his mother in a Dublin hospital six years before. We were asked to "write about the last real thing that happened to you."

My last real thing had occurred the week before, during my work in Seattle. I teach health policy to nursing students at the University of Washington. Together with colleagues in the Schools of Medicine and Dentistry, I help train groups of medical, nursing, and dental students in how to provide basic foot and dental care for homeless people. The week before my New York trip, we had done one of these Teeth and Toes clinics at Seattle's largest homeless shelter.

The shelter is in the downtown core of Seattle, at the bottom of the original Skid Road, which earned its name from the frontier town's cedar logs, public inebriates, and Gold Rush prostitutes, which all rolled downhill together into the mudflats and salt waters of Puget Sound. The front door to the shelter is at street level and opens onto a bare concrete staircase going up to the second floor, where the shelter services are located. Entering the building, I was hit by the smell of a horse stable, something hay-sweet mixed with urine and feces. The smell took me back to my work at the Cimmerian warehouse of the Richmond Street Center in Virginia, where I began my work with homeless people in the 1980s, and where I rolled down my own version of Skid Road and was homeless for six months. As this was not a time or a place I much wanted to revisit, the smell that hit me when I entered the Seattle shelter was revolting.

Later that evening, as I inspected various scars or open wounds on the homeless clients' feet, my mantra to them became, "What happened here?" Some people had simple replies, such as, "I was in a bad car accident a year ago." Other answers were more complex. One patient was a woman dressed in a stained orange T-shirt stretched over sagging, braless breasts, her short red hair flying away from florid, puffy cheeks. She stared at the ceiling while mumbling to herself, as if in prayer, her hands held in front of her neck, fluttering. I had the impression she was trying to catch hold of her exposed and scattered soul. Her only reply, while still looking at the ceiling and twitching her hands even faster, was, "I get nervous with too many questions."

Sitting next to her in a gray metal folding chair was a thin, middle-aged white man drawn into a frayed down vest, a military-style green cap on his head. He spit out at me, "It's a freak show here. I'm disabled, I've got depression, that's why I'm here with all these freaks!" Bitter, he was devouring himself in an endless loop, like an abortive Ouroboros.

The blown-apart woman and the spitting man are parts of myself I am still learning compassion for. They are parts of myself I would not likely meet were I a shoe buyer for Saks Fifth Avenue.

"What happened here?" is a question I asked myself as I spiraled into homelessness. At age twenty-five, I was a respectable Southern preacher's wife and a nurse, running a health care clinic for the homeless in downtown Richmond, my salary paid for by Catholic nuns. In a photo of me from this time, I'm kneeling on the floor of the clinic, my long straight hair falling in my face, and I'm washing the feet of a bearded Vietnam veteran homeless patient. I mostly worked alone in the clinic, tending to the health needs of thirty or more homeless patients each day for more than three years.

I have no photo of myself towards the end of those years, when I became a scarlet-lettered, depressed divorcee without a job, living in my car and in abandoned sheds. It was something out of a Southern Gothic tale, only it was real. I have no coherent story of this time, no map recording my journey, no facile answers to the question of what happened, only a mosaic of metaphors: rolling down Skid Road, falling into the rabbit hole, exposing my scattered soul, eating myself with rage—and flaming out. In retrospect, I see that my descent was partially caused by an extreme case of professional burnout, something nurses are especially prone to.

The term *professional burnout* comes from Graham Greene's novel *A Burnt-Out Case,* set in a colonial British Congo leprosy clinic staffed by an atheist physician and Catholic nuns as nurses. The physician explains that a burnt-out case is a leprosy patient whose disease has burned itself out: the patient no longer has active leprosy but has the scars such that he or she is unable to reenter normal life. In a conversation with the father superior of the village, the physician tells him of the issue of a leprophil: a person who is attracted to the suffering of lepers—who loves suffering and poverty and illness. It's a form of schadenfreude. The physician states that leprophil nurses "would rather wash the feet with their hair like the woman in the gospel than clean them with something more antiseptic." He likens leprophils to people who love and embrace poverty. The leprophil "makes for a bad nurse and ends by joining the patients." The physician tells the priest that a patient can detect when someone loves their disease, their poverty, their suffering, instead of loving them as a person.

Why are people drawn to work with the lepers, outcasts, and homeless of the world? Is it, as the priest states in Greene's novel, dangerous to ask what lies behind the desire to be of use, for we "might find some terrible things"?

The Christian charity piece fits for many of the people I've worked with, and it was what first drew me to my work with homeless and marginalized people. My father was a Presbyterian minister, as was my first husband. Albert Schweitzer had been my childhood idol. I had spent a year in seminary before becoming a nurse. I considered the work my religious calling.

Then there is humanist charity, for the nonreligious, a category I currently identify with. This virtuous work—or calling or vocation or zeal, whether religious or secular—can feed the Hungry Ghost ego. It can become one's identity; it can become addictive and destructive. I know this because I became my work, and through it, I became homeless.

Thinking of the various people I've worked with over the years—and thinking of my younger self—I've realized that many of us were working out our personal issues through our professional work. We were wounded in various ways, having battled alcohol and drug addictions, having survived childhoods of poverty or abuse. The latter was my own—at-the-time-unacknowledged—wound. Other people seemed drawn to the work out of guilt for a past life or action, and were doing penance for some self-assigned crime. For a few, that crime was having grown up with plenty.

In the narrative medicine workshop, there was an elegant, coolly detached young woman physician dressed in brocaded silk, with a large diamond-stud nose piercing and a diamond-encrusted gold watch on her slender wrist. She told us that she had been loaned an Italian villa to retreat to after finishing her PhD/MD, but once there, she grew restless, so she traveled to Bosnia to see real suffering, to visit the women who had survived systematic rape during the war. She told us this story in a crisply cut accent, while rearranging her silk scarf with her diamond and gold hand. I was struck by the incongruous juxtaposition of the diamonds, Italian villa, and PhD/MD degrees with seeking out the suffering of women in Bosnia.

Her in-your-face opulence was not something I was accustomed to seeing in Seattle, where REI polar fleece holds reign even among Microsoft and Amazon multimillionaires, and where it's considered ill-mannered to wear diamond-encrusted gold watches even if you can afford them. And thinking of someone that privileged and protected going on tourist jaunts to view poverty and suffering was repulsive. I recognized that I did not know this young woman; I had only met her three days before. She was clearly privileged, but perhaps she was not so protected. She likely had demons—a history of childhood sexual abuse or rape as a young woman, or something more benign like survivor's guilt or entitlement guilt—demons she was trying to face through her trip to Bosnia. Yet I had more difficulty finding compassion for her than for the obese woman with the scattered soul.

Perhaps that was because I was aware of—and uneasy with—parts of my own privilege, including the resources I had had to extract myself from poverty and homelessness, to deal with the wounds from my own childhood traumas, to obtain a good education and a decent-paying job, to purchase my own house, to pay for my son's college education—even the privilege of being able to afford this trip to New York City to attend this workshop, to be walking through these streets in Manhattan on a Sunday afternoon asking myself these questions.

There is the odd privilege, the luxury even, of having time and space for self-reflection. True reflection, soul-searching, is both a luxury and a danger. Such reflection should make us squirm, because it takes us to our shadowed places, to places of illness and pain, and to the sea-change of our existence.

On the southern edge of Central Park, I sat on an empty park bench to rest my foot. In front of me was the lovely fountain, titled *Abundance*, with the goddess Pomona holding an overflowing basket of fruit. To one side of the plaza was the shiny glass and steel Apple Store and on the other was the flag-festooned Plaza Hotel. All I carried was my frayed Thai Hill Tribe woven purse, but I felt like a bag lady sitting there on the park bench, surrounded by pigeons and in the midst of gilt. A willowy high-heeled young woman strolled past and glanced my way. In order to blend in and not appear so tattered, I pulled out my pen and notebook from my bag and began to write this essay. I could be an anthropologist! I could be a journalist! I could be an artsy angst-filled writer from Brooklyn!

But my foot throbbed and I saw that it was crusted with dark Manhattan grime. I had the image of my foot getting badly infected and having to be amputated. Sitting on the park bench on the edge of the Square of Abundance, I stopped writing, stopped asking questions which seemed only to lead to more questions, to questions which perhaps had no answers, or which perhaps had different answers depending on where I was along my journey.

I made it back to my New York seminary room later that Sunday. After I had washed my wounded foot thoroughly in the bathtub, I sat on my Spartan white bed and contemplated the split in my sole, deciding how best to help it heal. As I looked at the gaping eye-shaped hole weeping blush-colored salt water from my body, I memorized Percy Shelley's poem fragment "I love all waste." The poem was on a pocket card takeaway from the library exhibit. I realized that part of what draws me to my work is the expansive sense of connection with other people, with myself, and with the world. It is the fresh chance, every time, to find love and compassion for the obese woman with the scattered soul, for the man eating himself with anger, and even for myself walking with a wounded sole through Manhattan grime. It is the desire to connect with some wound deep inside and to seek soul health.

Two

Walk in My Shoes

People often ask themselves the right questions. Where they fail is in answering the questions they ask themselves.
—William Maxwell

On a cold, wet, blustery February afternoon, I sat observing shoe-buying rituals in the women's shoe section of the upscale Nordstrom store in downtown Seattle. Across the aisle from me was a red-haired young shoe saleswoman with a fluttery bright-blue silk scarf tied around her neck, retro airline stewardess style. She perched on a low metal stool in front of an elegantly dressed, middle-aged female customer. The customer sat ramrod straight, hands carefully crossed on one thigh, with a slightly bored demeanor. *Frosty with upper-crust breeding,* I noted as I sat slumped and smug in my chair.

"Oh, they're so darling! How do they feel?" the saleswoman asked.

"Good, but can I try them in black?"

"Of course! I'll be right back." The saleswoman jumped off her stool and disappeared into a back storage room.

I had spent the morning at a nearby women's homeless shelter as a nurse helping a group of ten medical and nursing students do foot care. Women soaked their feet in plastic dishpans of oatmeal-soaped water, while students sat on stools below them and washed their feet. I was at the shelter with a physician colleague from the university; together we supervised the students and intervened to provide any necessary treatment or referral for the patients. Providing something as intimate as foot care brings out stories in people. We encouraged the students to listen, to be able to hear, and perhaps to bear witness to the stories of homeless and marginalized people.

On my way into the Nordstrom store, I'd stopped to look at the bronze footprints of famous Seattleites scattered on the sidewalk. The largest pair was from Jim Whittaker, who climbed Mount Everest with his size twelve and a half, Vibram-soled, boot-clad feet. The smallest were the dainty high-heeled footprints of Mary Gates, famous for her philanthropy and for birthing Microsoft founder, billionaire, and global health guru Bill Gates. The footprints, or rather the shoe and boot prints, were next to large display windows filled with faceless plastic models wearing the latest shoe styles. The display mannequin pushed wooden carts, while outside on the sidewalk, homeless people pushed metal shopping carts. I stood at the store's threshold gazing at these displays and wondered: How many homeless people shuffle back and forth across these bronze footprints every day? Where in a city do homeless people leave their footprints?

As I walked into the shoe section of the store, I gazed at a pair of purple patent leather Doc Martens boots on a display table, wondering what sort of person would buy such garish shoes. I like shoes; I own a closetful of them. That day, I was wearing a pair of gray suede boots. They were the perfect combination of functionality (nonslippery soles, good for walking Seattle's hilly, rain-soaked streets) and style—hip without looking too young. Or at least I thought so. What did my boots say about me?

I reminded myself I wasn't there to shop. I was there to contemplate the meaning of shoes, and what it means to walk in another person's shoes. What better place to do that than in the Nordstrom shoe section during a sale?

Shoes are powerful markers of a person; shoes tend to hold the presence of the person who has worn them. In *The Year of Magical Thinking*, Joan Didion addresses this phenomenon. After the death of her husband from a massive heart attack, she finds herself holding on to his shoes. She writes, "I could not give away the rest of his shoes. I stood there for a moment, then realized why: he would need the shoes if he was to return. The recognition of the thought by no means eradicated the thought."

Several years ago, as I was sorting through my mother's closet after she died, I remembered this passage and finally understood it. More than any other item in my mother's bedroom—including the Estée Lauder perfume she wore every day—my mother's pair of cheap yellow canvas sneakers screamed of her existence. I filled bags to donate to Goodwill, but was compelled to hold on to her yellow shoes. She had worn them every winter while walking on the beach at Sanibel Island, stooped over, shelling. She had worn them while standing in her art studio, peering at a painting's progress. She had worn them after her once thin ankles puffed up with the by-products of cancer and of the poisonous cancer treatment. I finally got rid of her sneakers, but I threw them away instead of giving them to charity: I didn't want anyone else wearing my mother's shoes.

It was the red sneakers Essie was wearing that drew me to her at the women's shelter earlier that day. This was the second time in the past several months I had run into Essie at one of our foot care clinics. She wore an orange polyester shirt with a green chiffon scarf tied around her dreadlocks, a pink pleated skirt down to her ankles, and the red sneakers. She told me she only dressed in bright, Caribbean colors: "They keep me happy. I can't be all down in the dumps when I got these colors on." Essie had a perpetual and slightly crooked smile, the crookedness perhaps the residue of a stroke.

The women's shelter is located in a church basement in downtown Seattle near the main shopping district. It is a day shelter, a safe zone for women and children, that serves homeless and marginalized "near homeless" women, especially women dealing with domestic violence. The shelter has multiple case managers, social workers, and volunteer nurses who try to connect women with health, housing, and social services. The shelter workers lend the women a hand, bend an ear to hear their problems, offer a leg up the socioeconomic ladder, a toehold on life. Empathy is their main tool. Empathy is what we try to cultivate in our students.

Empathy is "feeling with" as opposed to "feeling for," which happens with at-arm's-length sympathy. "Walking in another person's shoes" is how empathy is most commonly described. But can we ever walk in another person's shoes? And is it always a good thing to try?

During my first interaction with Essie, she seemed so upbeat—frankly, normal—that I wondered why she was at the shelter as a client and not as a staff member. She must have sensed this, because she launched into a long story about her first day on the streets of Seattle. The how she got there to begin with part was hazy, as if becoming homeless came from some sort of blackout spell. But walking into the large downtown YWCA shelter for the first time seemed quite fresh in her memory. She described in vivid detail how she went in the front door of the YWCA and sat on a chair in the main room, only to have a woman immediately hiss at her, "That's my seat. You can't sit there!" Essie apologized and moved to another seemingly empty seat, only to have a different woman chase her off in a similar manner. An older woman took her aside and said, "You don't belong here. You should go up the street a ways to Mary's Place, where it's calmer and the women aren't as mean." So she did.

I enjoyed listening to Essie's stories, but the more she talked, the more cracks and inconsistencies I noticed, the more I imagined what sorts of traumas might have brought her to this place, and the more I emotionally held her at arm's length. I felt myself shrinking back; I even shifted my crouched position farther away from her. But I was simultaneously fascinated. What was wrong with her? The wanting to know more: was that empathy, or voyeurism, or schadenfreude, or a combination of all three?

Whenever I work with students in foot clinics, I remind them that we tend to be more empathetic towards people we know, people similar to us. That climbing the socioeconomic ladder often diminishes empathy. And that experiencing our own traumas can make us more empathetic to people who have experienced similar traumas. But being a wounded healer can also cause us to have more porous boundaries, which puts us at risk of losing our sense of self, our balance. I seldom am privy to the individual traumas of my students. I don't need to know this information. But I do need to know that they have access to resources that help them process—in positive ways—triggering events they may encounter. Participating in shelter-based foot clinics takes them out of the comforting, familiar walls of the hospital into more disturbing territory.

That morning at the women's shelter there had been a scab-faced, middle-aged white woman wearing a pork-pie hat, with tufts of green-dyed blond hair sticking out sideways. She kept using the shelter's phone on the wall, dialing, waiting a minute or so, slamming the receiver down with a loud "Aw

… damn you!" and aggressively pacing around the shelter, growling, "Get out of my way!" to random people—including me. I laughed softly: she was so preposterously angry it was funny. She reminded me of the *Angry Birds* computer game, and she resembled a deranged sandpiper with her rapid flitting back and forth across the room. I did not want to try to be in her shoes.

In the foot clinics we usually leave people's calluses alone and don't attempt to pumice them down or pare them away with a scalpel. Calluses are there for a reason; they are protective. Removing them would make the skin of the feet too vulnerable and expose them to worse traumas than those that caused the calluses in the first place.

The most delightful—and tender—foot clinic patient we had seen that morning was the petite three-year-old daughter of a young North African immigrant mother. The child pushed around a pink plastic toy shopping cart from the shelter's playroom, and she wore a dress, bright striped tights, black Mary Janes, and a huge pink feather boa around her neck. She came and sat on a metal folding chair while one of the students washed her mother's feet. The little girl wanted her own feet to be given the same attention, so her mother removed her shoes and tights. Baby toes! So cute!

I asked her mother for permission to photograph just her daughter's feet. I wanted to capture some of the freshness and innocence of those baby toes in the room full of hardened, scarred, bitter women. I wanted to scoop her up and protect her from becoming like these women, to keep her from the traumas, the abuses of the world. But, of course, I knew I couldn't do that. It made me sad to watch her toes curl up in delight as she splashed her feet in the basin of soapy water.

Advertisers use a form of empathy to sell things. Like shoes. The red-haired shoe saleswoman at Nordstrom was "feeling-into" her haughty female customer, intuiting what would flatter her into buying an expensive pair of shoes. I sat in the Nordstrom shoe section that day in February long enough to see that it worked: this particular customer bought those shoes along with two more pairs in other colors. The saleswoman picked up the shoes the customer had worn into the store and said, "We'll just send these back to Chanel for resoling."

When I heard this part of their conversation, I sighed and repositioned myself in the chair. I resisted the urge to stand up and tell them about the eight-year-old girl in the shelter that morning with badly blistered and macerated feet from wearing a pair of fake and ill-fitting leather boots—the only shoes she owned. Wearing the mantle of self-righteousness as if it were a hair shirt is something I have learned to be aware of and to shrug off before it sticks to me. That day in Nordstrom, I chose to distract myself from my discomfiting tangle of thoughts and emotions by taking photographs of the rows and rows of bright and shiny shoes.

Who goes to the United States Holocaust Memorial Museum in Washington, DC, and isn't forever haunted by its display of a roomful of shoes? You look at the monstrous pile of shoes towering above your head. You realize what the shoes represent. You register that without that thick pane of glass separating you from them, the shoes would suffocate you. The shoes smell faintly of rubber and of musty, moldering leather. The collective smell of the shoes from the concentration camps seeps over the top of the glass wall and enters your own body.

There are men's ankle-high lace-up work boots, children's simple ankle boots, Mary Jane strapped little girl's shoes, and fancy women's dress shoes, some with dulled rhinestones on the straps. The display placard explains that most of the people taken to the camps wore their finest shoes because they were told they were being relocated to a better place.

Mixed in with the fancier shoes are ones with worn-through soles and battered leather. Perhaps these belonged to homeless people and street prostitutes who were rounded up and sent to concentration camps along with Jews and Gypsies and disabled people.

The hardest to look at are the tiny infant shoes tossed in with all the rest. These shoes had been white but are now ashen with age.

The Holocaust Museum's shoe display came back to me unexpectedly when I worked at the King County Juvenile Detention Center in Seattle. I wasn't there to provide health care or foot care, but rather to help the young people write poetry. During orientation, we were taken on a tour of the facility, starting with the intake unit, a portion of the detention facility with a separate entrance through which the police officers escort young detainees. A central glass-enclosed office for the intake officers dominates the unit. We were admonished never to call them guards and were forcefully corrected if we slipped. The term *guard* was beneath them somehow—because officers are better educated than guards? I didn't quite understand why. But juvenile detention—or "juvie" for short, although we were admonished never to call it juvie—is not a place to question much of anything, even if you are an adult.

The morning we walked through the unit, a male officer sat at a desk behind the glass partition. He was chatting with a female officer sitting next to him. Snatches of their conversation floated out to me.

"I don't get it. In lesbian sex there's got to be one that's the guy, right?" the male officer asked, gesticulating wildly with both hands.

The female guard laughed nervously, glanced our way, and said, "Don't ask me! I'm surely not no lesbian!"

Outside the glassed-in office, a huge officer with a shaved head was describing his high-tech toys to us: the fingerprint scanner and the mug-shot camera.

"Digital fingerprints we take of all ten fingers starting with number one, the right thumb, like this. Then number two, right index finger, all the way over to number ten, the left pinky finger. And then we take their headshots. The headshots are very important. They can't wear nothing on their heads and they can't smile."

Why couldn't the young people smile? Was it just part of intimidation, psychological control, or to keep them uniform for lineups so victims could identify their perpetrators? I was already too intimidated by the culture of the place to be able to ask.

"But this here is what can really prove they did it or not." The officer waved a giant Q-tip over his head. He explained that they take cheek swabs from young people charged with sex crimes or other violent crimes, label the samples, and place them in a locked black metal box, marked DNA, for processing by the crime laboratory.

I had been glancing discreetly behind me during his presentation. A petite, ponytailed African American girl was being processed for intake. She appeared to be approximately thirteen and wore tight-fitting jeans, a shiny pink shirt, and bright-pink dangly earrings with a matching necklace. Her earrings and necklace looked like Barbie-doll paste jewelry. A female officer ordered her to remove all her clothes, except her underwear, and to put on a pair of what resembled dark-blue hospital scrubs—a loose-fitting V-neck tunic shirt and drawstring pants.

Beneath the curtain, I could see the girl untie her glittery pink high-tops. I almost expected them to contain those obnoxious flashing LED lights in the soles. They screamed little girl. I watched her replace her shoes with the detention-issued ankle-high white socks and thick blue rubber flip-flops.

As the bald officer droned on about how important his job was, I saw the female officer roughly scoop up the girl's belongings—including the pink high-tops—and toss them into a large zippered black garment bag that looked like the body bags we use in hospitals to dispose of dead patients. This is when I thought of the shoe room at the United States Holocaust Memorial Museum. Intellectually, I knew they weren't the same, but in that moment, they were similar enough to make me nauseous. I willed myself not to look away as the officer wrote the girl's name on the label and took the bag to a storage rack on the other side of the room.

Time of death, I thought, and found myself looking around for a clock to check the time. Clearly, I'd been watching too many *ER* episodes. There were four digital clocks scattered on the walls in the intake unit and out in the hallway. I looked at them and realized that they had all stopped at 08:52:20. The clocks stayed at 08:52:20 for the four months I worked there.

I should have walked out of juvenile detention that day and never returned. But I wanted to tough it out. I had spent most of my life working with homeless, marginalized, and prostituted teens, providing them with primary health care. I had lived through my own version of childhood trauma, and as a young adult had spiraled into deep depression and home-lessness. But I had never spent time in juvie or in jail. Many of the young people I worked with had been in various juvenile detention units around the country, so I wanted to know more of what they experienced.

In *The Empathy Exams*, Leslie Jamison describes her work as a medical actor for standardized patient exams at a medical school. After each mock exam, she evaluates the medical student on various attributes, including "voiced empathy." Did they ask permission before pressing a stethoscope to her chest? Did they respond with something close to "That must be really hard" when she revealed a painful part of her past history? Jamison describes empathy as "a penetration, a kind of travel. It suggests you enter another person's pain as you'd enter another country, through immigration and customs, border crossing by way of query: *What grows where you are? What are the laws? What animals graze there?*"

The building that houses the King County Juvenile Detention Center is old, squat, and industrial-looking. There are layers of security to pass through: a metal detector and X-ray machine at the front entrance, small lockers to store your belongings, a guard behind glass who collects your driver's license, and then the long wait before being asked to stand inside a glass-walled automatic double-door holding tank between the waiting room and the inner sanctum of juvenile detention. I was never sure of the purpose of the holding tank. It felt claustrophobic, like being inside an airport body scanner or an MRI machine.

Once inside, you are greeted by the sound of heavy metal doors slamming and the clinking of the large rings of keys each officer wears chained to his or her waist. An oily slime covers every surface. Stale dust motes float in the air along with the smell of bleach and institutional food. The stained concrete floors are littered with wads of old chewing gum turned white, brittle, and flat—gum containing all those strands of DNA, no cheek-swabs required. Along the windowless hallways, groups of young detainees walk in single file flush against the walls, their hands clasped behind their backs, heads down, not talking. These are the rules. The *thwack, thwack, thwack* of their heavy rubber flip-flops echoes through the cavernous hallways.

We wrote poems with the young people, or rather, we wrote poems *for* the young people. Like the professional letter writers of the past who wrote letters for illiterate or semiliterate people, we sat on stone benches across tables from young detainees and pried words and emotions from them. Sometimes they knew what they wanted to write about—typically flowery love letters by the young women and gang brotherhood poems by the young men. Missing their families. Asking their mothers for forgiveness for causing them such grief. Asking forgiveness from the victims of their crimes. Admonishing their little brothers and sisters not to follow in their footsteps.

This is how a love letter should be; *this* is how a poem should be: we altered their words, their sentences, their metaphors, trying to make them fit our notion of cathartic poetry. We five white adults who could walk out of juvie at the end of the day, see trees, see our families, sleep in our own beds, go to work the next day at our well-paying jobs—wear our own shoes. But I kept returning to juvie, kept prying that angst-filled poetry from the young people. We had an unwritten code: the more the angst, the deeper the pain, the better the poem.

"Empathy can be a story you tell yourself about what it must be like to be that other person; but its lack can also arise from narrative, about why the sufferer deserved it, or why that person or those people have nothing to do with you," writes Rebecca Solnit in *The Faraway Nearby*. She points out that people can be encouraged to distance themselves from marginalized people, but then that distancing or dissociation or deadening causes us to be "stranded in the islands of ourselves." Using the young people in juvie to write our own versions of what we thought their stories should be, I began to feel more distant from them—and from myself.

But I simultaneously began to feel overly close to them, to their situation. At night, I startled awake from nightmares of being locked inside juvie, mute, unable to scream for help or to escape.

It was probably inevitable that one day I would be sitting at a table beside the girl I had seen wearing glittery pink high-tops, serving as her scribe. She walked in, not talking, glanced furtively around the room at the available tables, and sat across from me. In response to my questions, she told me she had just turned fourteen. Then, through her poem that I wrote on a yellow legal pad, she began to talk. Her story was a familiar one: absent father presumed dead from drugs. Mother dead from drugs. Sexually abused as a child by her mother's live-in boyfriend. Multiple foster home placements from which she ran away. Lured into street prostitution at age twelve by her older boyfriend who was really her pimp. This was her eighth time in juvie, and she said it casually as if it were a minor irritation. The judges often sentence girls for time in juvie as a way to get them off the streets, into relative safety, and to connect them with services like counseling, health care, and housing. It hadn't been working for her, but then, at least she was still alive. Writing her poem was like diving off a cliff into an open, festering cesspool.

The cesspool got even murkier: my next poetry-writing session that day was with a seventeen-year-old African American male. He sat next to me as I helped him write poetry about the remorse he felt over pimping young girls.

Perhaps it was real remorse or perhaps just a rehearsal for what his lawyer and the judge wanted to hear. As I tried to reach for at least some stirring of empathy, to push past the anger and disgust I felt for who he was, for what he had done, I only felt profoundly sad. I had the urge to curl up on the floor beneath the table, my face pressed to the dried wads of chewing gum, and listen to the murmuring strands of DNA spinning webbed tales of trauma—and of survival.

At the end of the day, we typed their poetry and printed out copies, some pages to file away for the poetry program to sell as chapbooks, and others to give to the youths who had ostensibly written them. We trudged down the hallway to their individual rooms. The only personal items young people could have in their cells were Bibles and the pages of their poems. No pens or pencils, no paper clips or even staples: all could be used as weapons against themselves or other people.

The guard told me that the pink high-top girl was in the clinic and to just slide her poems under her door. I peeked inside the window and saw a tiny, barren room with a metal-platform twin bed and a slit of a barred window near the ceiling. In a corner of the room near the door, there was a sink, a stainless steel seatless toilet, and a scratched shiny plate of metal in lieu of a mirror.

Going into the boys' unit to find the seventeen-year-old, I noticed they had to leave their flip-flops outside their doors. I found his room and knocked gently, saying that I had his poems. He responded with a "yeah, okay" before I looked in the window to see him lying on his bed, arms behind his head, staring up at the whitewashed ceiling. In that pose he looked incredibly young and vulnerable.

I moved the shoes aside, pushed his poems under the door, then gave him a thumbs up and a "Good job, take care of yourself" through the window. He smiled, said, "Thanks," and swung his legs out of bed to retrieve the poems.

Looking at those blue flip-flops in front of the doors of the juvie cells, I knew I could never walk in their shoes. And the young people: would they even want me to try? Do people on the receiving end of empathy always experience it as a good thing? Or do they sometimes see it as prying, as pity?

I quit my volunteer job at juvie soon after. The clocks remained stuck at

08:52:20. It was as if I had never been there. The words—the real words—of both the pink high-top girl and the young male pimp remain etched in my memory. Their words combine and reform into questions: What did we all do to allow this to happen? To be okay with locking young people in such a dismal place? Okay with thinking that prying poetry from them somehow made it all more palatable?

I still see Essie and the angry bird woman at the women's shelter when I take students to do foot clinics. I recognize more of myself in the angry woman, so I no longer laugh at her flitting rage. I now find delight not only in Essie's brightly garish clothing, but also in her behavioral quirks and crooked smile.

And the haughty shoe buyer at Nordstrom? I ask myself why I thought it was okay to sit at a distance, coolly observing, jotting down notes, as if she were a faceless mannequin, and to smugly judge her shoe-buying behavior. We all have some aspect of the Hungry Ghost emptiness we attempt to feed. I knew I was making assumptions about this woman. Perhaps I envied her—not her apparent discretionary income, but her apparent ability to distance herself from the suffering of people right outside the Nordstrom doors. And I wondered: if she had children or a spouse to clean her closet after her death, would they know which shoes screamed of her existence?

That's the thing about empathy: reaching for empathy for a person we find distasteful requires seeing some of ourselves in them; seeing our common humanity; seeing and forgiving our own distasteful parts; walking—carefully, compassionately, calluses and all—in our own shoes.

Three

Witness: On Seeing

Bearing witness constitutes a specific form of collective remembering …
—Barbie Zelizer

Christchurch, New Zealand. Central Business District Red Zone, January 2014.

"Witness a city in transformation," proclaims the New York Times article "52 Places to Go in 2014." It's referring to Christchurch, listed as the number-two top place to visit. The article is accompanied by a photograph of the stained glass window in the newly constructed Cardboard Cathedral in downtown Christchurch.

I have arrived in the Central Business District (CBD) knowing almost nothing of Christchurch except that it is still in the process of rebuilding three years after two large earthquakes destroyed most of its downtown core. I'm teaching environmental and community health to a group of sixteen undergraduate university students on a three-month-long study abroad program. We flew into Christchurch yesterday, and we're staying at an agricultural college on the outskirts of town. Today, a sunny summer Sunday, we've taken the city bus into the CBD to look around and to get our bearings.

We stumble off the bus at the central bus depot and gaze at several blocks' worth of concrete rubble. The air we breathe smells of acerbic mortar mixed with the salt tang of the nearby Pacific. We walk towards what our map tells us is the center of town. The first building we encounter is a destroyed but still standing three-story parking garage. Its exit sign dangles by a thin wire. Swallows swoop in and out. Across the street is a tall brick façade of an old building, now propped up by towering stacks of brightly colored shipping containers held in place with steel cables. Curving pathways of orange safety cones and temporary chain-link fences mark safe and unsafe places to walk. The only sounds I hear are the cries of birds mingled with the rumbling bus engine behind me. At first I hesitate, then I pull my camera from my bag and begin taking photographs.

Once I start taking photographs, I can't stop. Banners on streetlights depicting a bright, colorful, intact city. A cocktail lounge, Showgirls neon sign (unlit) in a partially boarded-up window of an otherwise destroyed building. Large painted graffiti and artwork murals adorning exteriors of still-standing buildings. Lovely old architectural details, such as carved stone arches and columns, and even intact stained glass windows in partial walls. More stacks of shipping containers. More steel cables. Charred remains of stores and apartment buildings. Piles of mangled wire and iron rebar. Industrial-sized Dumpsters full of building debris. A Starbucks store at street level with a boarded-up door and "OK. TFI Clear. 26/2" written in orange paint across its windows: the store was searched for dead people four days after the most destructive earthquake. Orange cranes. Steel supporting struts holding up stone building façades as if they're stage props. Long stretches of dusty, empty lots. For Sale signs on dusty, empty lots. For Sale or Lease signs on shipping containers. A large, exposed concrete basement of a building: On one of its walls is a cubbyhole filled with stacks of phone books, their yellow pages ruffled and faded. A tattered black backpack is splayed on the ground beneath.

Seagulls cry and fly in and out of the ruins. Tufts of grass and yellow and orange flowers sprout from broken windowsills. *Over your cities grass will grow*—a vaguely Biblical quote—comes to me within the memory of an art installation by one of my favorite artists, Anselm Kiefer. Kiefer grew up in post–World War II Germany. As a child, he played in the ruins of his city—ruins that have haunted his art ever since.

Turning a corner, we hear hymns being sung in a church set up inside a shipping container. In front of the church are empty white painted chairs of all sizes and descriptions: desk chairs, bar stools, lawn chairs, stuffed lounge chairs, folding chairs, rocking chairs, children's chairs, director's canvas chairs, infant car seats, infant high chairs, and wheelchairs. *What are they?* I wonder. *Outdoor seating for a church service?* One of my students reads the sign explaining that this is *Reflection of Loss of Lives, Livelihood and Living in Neighborhood,* an art installation by Peter Majendie to memorialize the 185 people who died in the earthquake: 185 chairs, each representing the individual killed. "The installation is temporary—as is life," the artist states. The sign invites us to sit quietly in a chair to which we are drawn. I sit in a desk chair next to a wheelchair and consider what terror it must have been for an elderly or disabled person to be trapped and killed by the earthquake. I pull my hat tighter to shield my face from the hot sun. Then I take many photographs of the chairs. Of individual chairs. Of my students sitting in chairs. The chairs are witnesses; the chairs are funerary monuments. It occurs to me that the vast majority of chairs are desk chairs, as if from a school. I wonder what this means.

We cross the street to yet another empty lot, this one surrounded by tall chain-link fencing decorated by scattered offerings: withered bouquets of flowers, bits of ribbon, even pipe cleaners spelling out people's names. A small placard affixed to the fence tells us this was the site of the CTV—Canterbury Television—building, a six-story building that pancaked and burned in the earthquake, killing 115 people. The CTV building housed a television headquarters, an English as a second language school, a medical clinic, and a nursing school. Students were the bulk of the casualties.

Next to the CTV lot is the Cardboard Cathedral, a large white A-frame constructed from reinforced cardboard packing tubes, with eight shipping containers forming the two long sides. Inside, it feels spacious, clean, and light-filled, with everything made of cardboard, even a large cross and pulpit in the front of the church. The only color comes from the triangle-shaped stained glass window over the entrance at the back of the cathedral. Each of the smaller triangles of colored glass—red, yellow, green, blue, and white—contains only fractured bits of images, such as wings and halos, faces, and hands held in prayer.

The images come from a high-resolution photograph of the now destroyed rose window in the Gothic Revival stone Christchurch Cathedral that had stood for a century and a half nearby in the town square. The circular window had been the city's main icon. The first earthquake, on September 4, 2010, spared the window, and people talked of it as a miracle and a symbol of the resilience of their city. But the second earthquake, on February 22, 2011, destroyed the window and the cathedral, along with many people's hope. Shigeru Ban, the Japanese architect who designed the

Cardboard Cathedral, incorporated fractured bits of the rose window into his stained glass window, taking something that was ruined, reconfiguring it, and making it into something new and beautiful.

Entering the town square, I first see the gray mounds of what is left of the old Christchurch Cathedral. I take several photographs. Then, near me in the square, I notice a homeless young man in a wheelchair. He's a deeply tanned white man who looks to be in his early twenties, and he is wearing layers of clothes and a coat on this warm summer day. Tied to the back of his wheelchair is a duffel bag and a dirty rolled-up sleeping bag. As I pretend to look at other buildings in the square, I see two teenage girls, equally dirty and disheveled, walk up and sit on a bench next to the young man. From the tone and content of their conversation, it's apparent they are all friends: street friends, street family. They are homeless rough sleepers in the British parlance of New Zealand, or "streeties" in the blunt Kiwi slang. I had read that over half of New Zealand's homeless population was under the age of twenty-five, and that the earthquakes greatly increased the overall number of homeless people. I suddenly realize that the cordoned-off and condemned buildings I have been photographing are likely the temporary homes or "squats" of the homeless young people beside me.

Behind them, I see a lovely old ornate brick building. It appears to be some sort of government building and is intact, but has boarded-up windows and is fenced off. Then I look at its clock tower and notice that the clocks have lost their hands. Time stops here. How fitting for the sense of suspended, distorted, thickened time I feel I have unwittingly entered. My students have scattered like pigeons across the square. Feeling vaguely dizzy, I sit on a bench in the shade of a large tree.

I'd had no idea we could just casually walk through all of this. I'd had no idea of how fresh the destruction would seem and how little recovery we would see. I am overwhelmed by the disaster tourism—*thanatourism*—we seem to be doing. The disaster tourism I am participating in. Taking photographs, telling myself the photographs are for teaching, but feeling uncomfortable, as if I were a voyeur at the site of a huge, bloody car crash—detached, clicking away, with the camera lens between me and the destruction. I can carry the images home and do whatever I want with them. It occurs to me that I'm not even sure what I'm seeing, what the camera is seeing, what I've included and what I've left out of the photographs. What stories, what fractured bits of stories, will they contain? And what am I supposed to do with these stories?

I try to convince myself it's okay to take photographs because no one lives here anymore, not in the CBD Red Zone that's been condemned by the government. It's not like I'm taking photographs of dead bodies. But I know that people were injured and died in these crumbling buildings and rubble-strewn streets. And now I realize that people like these homeless teenagers still live amidst the ruins. This is their home. The realization makes me squirm.

I become lost in a spiral of questions: What is the human fascination with the macabre? Is it schadenfreude? Is it, as Susan Sontag wrote in *On Photography*, "the feeling of being exempt from calamity"—from this tragedy, this trauma, this crime, this violence that has happened to someone else, not to me? Is it sublime fear, the most elemental of emotions, that draws us in, staring, transfixed in these still-blazing headlights?

My students begin to flock back around me, bringing me out of my reverie. I don't share what I've been thinking with the students; my thoughts are too random, unformed, and tangled with personal preoccupations and raw emotion. We resume our odd and melancholy community walkabout and head to an art museum highlighted on the tourist map. Artists and writers are cultural and spiritual first responders in a disaster: they aid in the attempt to make meaning out of catastrophe and chaos, to find ways to not only survive but also thrive in the midst of adversity. They point the way to healing, to the melding of remembrance and forgiveness, to endurance.

We come to a series of shipping containers set on yet another dusty, empty lot. There's an abstract, brightly painted smiling face on the outside of one of the containers, along with the sign "Christchurch Art Gallery at Art Box." Inside is an interactive video installation called *Bodytok Quintet* by the New Zealand artist Phil Dadson. Dadson made up the word *bodytok* from a Melanesian pidgin word, *toktok*, which means "to have a conversation." The installation is a series of video recordings of ordinary people making eccentric preverbal, prelingual sounds with various parts of their bodies: belly drumming, skin slapping, finger cracking, and tongue clicking. These are the elemental building blocks of communication—the primal first language. Each video recording is interactive. It starts and speeds up the closer you move towards the screen, then slows down and becomes a framed portrait of the person as you move away. The video recordings interact with your body, with your presence. Someone must be there to listen and to hear, to observe and to see—to witness.

As I watch, listen, and interact with these video recordings, and observe my students doing the same, I wonder if this is how people communicate during and immediately after earthquakes. Are gestures and body sounds the main components of communication when trauma overwhelms coherent language, coherent narrative? And are these elements of narrative sufficient to bear witness to experience?

After walking through the Christchurch earthquake destruction, I sought out stories from people who had lived through the quakes. I listened for people's stories while riding the city bus and while sitting in coffee shops. People used the term "quake brain" to describe their fuzzy thinking, the indecision, bewilderment, disbelief, and exhaustion that accompanied the prolonged recovery efforts. I heard people liken it to the oozing gray lique-faction continuing to complicate the rebuilding of their city. Liquefaction, where once stable soil becomes swamp mud, quicksand, swallowing solid things like buildings, cars, or people.

"If the English language had a word for the false sense of familiarity you feel when you encounter in real life the situation you've often seen onscreen, I'd use it here," writes Christchurch resident Philip Armstrong in his *Landfall* essay "On Tenuous Grounds." From Armstrong, I learn that the February Christchurch earthquake killed tourists who were walking through the CBD taking photographs. I wonder what images their cameras contained, and if any of their photographs were of the destruction from the previous earthquake. I am reminded of what Roland Barthes points out in *Camera Lucida*, that cameras are "clocks for seeing," and photographic images are themselves a form of mortality, proof of time passing.

"While photographing subjects do not intentionally contribute to, alter, or seek to alter or influence events."

This statement is part of the code of ethics for the National Press Photographers Association. It is listed number five, right after "Treat all sub-jects with dignity and respect," calling out a special consideration to be given to vulnerable subjects. This is part of the official written code that underlies the unwritten code of conduct which most professional photographers and visual journalists hold themselves to.

This seems like such a banal statement. How can any grounded, empathetic human live up to this code of ethics? And aren't they—aren't I—by the very act of observing, of taking photographs, turned into a witness at some level, whether intended or not?

The rules and professional boundaries of journalism and photojournalism are meant to keep people from getting personally involved, because that diminishes the supposed objective gaze—as if such a thing were even possible. These rules are, of course, similar for health care professionals in terms of maintaining healthy personal boundaries with patients. Such rules are really meant to protect the photographer, the professional, because bearing the weight of witnessing can become too much. Here, I am reminded of Kevin Carter, the white South African photographer who shot the haunting photograph of the vulture seemingly about to eat a starving child in Africa. He was criticized for pausing to photograph instead of helping the child. And the American photographer Diane Arbus who sought out and captured in photographs the maimed, the tortured, the grotesque. She wasn't a photojournalist per se, but she was criticized for staying within the safety of the privileged, and gazing dispassionately at the Other. Both Carter and Arbus killed themselves. Was it the criticism, the photographs, or their peculiar twists on observing and witnessing that led them to such despair?

The Christchurch story is not my story, but then it became part of my story. I was not there as a detached observer or as a camera-wielding tourist—I was there, albeit unwittingly, as a witness. I had to declare my own stake in what I saw, in what I experienced.

Traumas have a way of unearthing partially buried relics of previous traumas. My students had a difficult time processing the destruction and the lack of progress in recovery efforts. As did I. But I was responsible for their health and well-being during the program, so I spent time talking with them as a group and individually. Most of the students made it through this difficult time, but one student decided to return to her family in Seattle.

Since I process emotional events through writing, I wrote a blog post, opening with this:

Clearly, I was an Ugly American Tourist/Professor stumbling (unprepared) into the Red Zone of Christchurch yesterday. But I wasn't prepared for the magnitude of the still-raw destruction in the downtown core. How long does it take to clean up a city after a major disaster? More than three years? That is what I thought—and still think—although I recognize I really know very little about the politics and psyche of this country I am visiting. … But I keep asking myself, "Why are we here?" Are we inadvertently participating in trauma tourism—also called disaster tourism, dark tourism, thanatourism? In downtown Christchurch, they even have those very British double-decker sightseeing buses labeled Red Zone Tours. At least we didn't pay to ride on one of those, but is it even worse to have walked around taking photos of destruction, peering into windows of what people left behind when they fled?

I also wasn't prepared for the response to my blog post. Responses, mainly from residents of Christchurch, started pouring in. One of the first comments was this:

Cycling to school through the residential red zone, to see buses of tourists taking photos is quite disturbing. Oh, to have a day where I see no reminders of the quakes. To have a "normal" day would be amazing.

There were many people who voiced anger and frustration at the lack of adequate assistance from the New Zealand government and from insurance companies. Several small business owners from Christchurch—including a jeweler who sold "wee Earthquake damaged house charms" for bracelets, depicting crumbled houses—defended their actions as trying to stay afloat financially. And many other people wrote sentiments such as, "I'm glad you came and brought your students. It makes us feel less isolated." But the following comment stands out as the most poignant:

Please tell others to come and be a part of our collective mess. Sitting side-by-side with all the pain, loss, and suffering is beauty and vibrant community and the precious gift of being alive.

I do use many of the Christchurch photographs in my teaching about community health and community resilience. When I look again at the photographs, I see things I missed when I was there. Perhaps, in part, because of the comments to my blog post, I now notice all the signs of regrowth, not just the volunteer yellow and orange flowers sprouting up, but all the other fun, creative things amidst the rubble. Like the dorky-sounding Dance-O-Mat that my students discovered and danced on for several hours in the bright sunshine, alongside young Christchurch children who laughed and pranced as children should. And in many of the photographs, I see my reflection in remnants of glass in the destroyed buildings that were the object of my gaze.

Four

Witness: On Telling

Telling stories is as basic to human beings as eating. More so, in fact, for while food makes us live, stories are what make our lives worth living.
—Richard Kearney

When trauma, illness, or injury occurs, a common human response is to want to tell the story of it, and to reach out for the stories of others who have had similar experiences, yet found ways to recover, or at least to make peace with what happened. Trauma is an experience that threatens our physical and emotional well-being and causes fear and a sense of helplessness. Trauma changes how we understand our world and ourselves. We seek ways to create a coherent narrative out of trauma, illness, or injury: the "tick"—this happened—which causes the expectation of the "tock"—then that happened. Plotting presupposes and requires an end, just as the plot of our lives requires death. Narrative in some form—spoken, written, or visual—organizes human ways of knowing and of remembering the past.

Sociologist Arthur W. Frank, in his book *The Wounded Storyteller*, presents a typology of illness stories. Frank contends that there is a universal urge for ill or injured persons to tell their stories, to change the passivity of being a victim of fate into the activity of what the ill or injured person did in response to the trauma. He points out that the sharing of these illness stories can be of healing benefit to both the teller and the listener. Being seriously injured or ill threatens us; it becomes a form of trauma. These types of events force us to confront our own mortality, to redraw our personal maps, to rethink our destinations. Stories we tell ourselves and others are ways of redrawing these maps and of recalibrating our destinations.

Serious illness or injury—what Frank calls "deep illness"—disrupts our memory. It makes us, at least temporarily, become disoriented and lose our way. Painful bodily, psychic, and spiritual memories are so threatening that they can distort past, present, and future. The making and telling of our stories help us reconstitute self and memory. But this making and telling of stories always presupposes an audience—even if we are our own audience: story happens within a social context, and story takes on social functions.

According to Frank, one of the most common illness narratives is the restitution story: I was healthy, then I became ill or injured, but now I'm healthy again. These are the illness stories that are most strongly sanctioned by our society and institutions. They are the illness story plotlines conveyed in get-well cards. We all want the healthy, functioning, predictable, and seemingly safe body back again. At the community level, this is the illness story told by the post–Hurricane Katrina New Orleans Mardi Gras celebration and the Boston Strong campaign after the marathon bombings.

The restitution storyline is the type used in those somewhat saccharine personal testimonial fundraising efforts launched by various helping agencies, including hospitals. They are easily digestible sound bites of stories: "Suzie O had a life-threatening automobile accident that left her temporarily paralyzed, but with the excellent medical care of our hospital, she is walking again." But, as Frank points out, restitution stories aren't an individual's own illness story, because they are prescripted and prescribed, part of the larger metanarrative of societal expectations.

What would it mean if I were to tell you a story with the following plot summary?

> I had a reasonably happy childhood, but as a young adult I spiraled into things I shouldn't have, including into abusive relationships and into homelessness. Then, with help from friends and family and institutions, I got on my feet again, and now I am fine. I am a homeowner. I have raised two well-adjusted children. I am a tenured professor. For the past twenty years I have been in a healthy long-term relationship. I could be the poster child for the National Alliance to End Homelessness.

And what would this version of my story mean for people who have not been able to "overcome" or "get well" from homelessness and poverty and abusive relationships? Doesn't this version of my story convey the message "If I can do it, so can they; therefore, what's wrong with them?" But for many years, this is the illness narrative I tried to tell myself, and that I told to other people. The narrative felt safe—the easy way out; it also rang false in the telling. I always wanted to blurt out at the end, *But really, that's not what happened.* I didn't actually say that because I wasn't sure what came next. I wasn't sure how to tell a different version of my story.

The second type of illness narrative, according to Frank, is the familiar quest narrative. We often have a rigid, scripted notion of what a good, linear, satisfying, and effective quest story arc should be. It is usually the hero slaying demons and dragons of some sort, and emerging at the end triumphant and transformed, and even stronger and more handsome. The feminist version of the quest narrative has the young woman descending into the Underworld, wearing a lot of jewelry (and perhaps fancy shoes) as armor and for buying her way out of difficult circumstances, and then emerging again into the light and the land of the living much wiser and more beautiful—although with much less jewelry and perhaps also barefoot and pregnant. These are the New Age, Joseph Campbell–like, *you are the hero or heroine of your own story* stories.

In his book, Frank implies that the quest narrative is the privileged way to go; it is the higher-order illness narrative. Our society seems to agree with him, with its myriad personal storytelling projects, memoirs, novels, confessional-type television talk shows, tabloid articles, movie scripts, and narrative therapies. We want soft-focus Hallmark moments that make us feel all warm and cozy inside.

So here is the quest illness narrative version of my story—with a feminist slant:

My father was a Presbyterian minister. I had a reasonably happy childhood until age fourteen, when I had a string of serious illnesses including red measles, followed by panic attacks and a deep depression, followed by anorexia. My parents admonished me to use the illnesses as a dark night of the soul, as a message to get right with God. I tried that. After college, I married a soon-to-be Presbyterian minister, hoping that by "finding religion" I could cure myself. But I fell back into a depression after the birth of my first child. Depression was my Underworld. I had an affair with a much older—and, as it turned out, abusive—man, and lost my job, home, and family, more or less in that order.

My turning point came through swimming. Despite living in my car for a time, I had access to a YMCA gym where I showered and swam miles each day. Determined to face one of my deepest fears, I trained for and competed in the Chesapeake Bay Bridge Race: four and a half miles of cold, dark, fast-moving water between Annapolis, Maryland, and the Eastern Shore of Virginia. I had 12 percent body fat. For the Bay Bridge race, I wore a one-piece racing suit with a neoprene vest partial wet suit. I wore no jewelry since I was convinced it would attract sharks.

Halfway through the race, my hands and feet went numb. When I turned my head to the side for a breath, through foggy goggles I saw the looming pillars of the bridge and the black race number written on my left bicep. I hallucinated that the bridge was a warship and that the black number on my arm was a Nazi concentration camp number—a concentration camp from which I was escaping. I realized I had hypothermia, so I kicked harder in order to get to warmer water.

I finished the race. This experience gave me the strength to kick like hell, get myself out of the suffocating South, out of the abusive relationship, out of homelessness. I emerged from this deep illness stronger, transformed—a wounded healer. I experienced a redemptive rebirth through the trials of homelessness and its attendant ills. I emerged transformed and resilient. I could write a best-selling memoir and have a Hallmark movie made of my life.

This is the version of my story I held on to—like a safety kayak—for many years. I wrote a book manuscript using this version of my story. Decades after I had survived these chapters of my life, I had this story published and made public. But I did this only after my career was well established, my children were grown, and my parents were deceased. Because it was a dangerous story; it was a disruptive story. This story could derail my career and complicate, if not end, my personal relationships.

Yet the more I lived with this story, the more I realized that it wasn't true—not that the events didn't happen, but I did not experience them in the simple Aristotelian plotline way that I was retelling them. This version is too sanitized, too streamlined; it doesn't dip into the murky depths of emotions, of power dynamics, of what I was experiencing internally at the time, or of how I remember it now.

The least desirable illness narratives, according to Frank, are what he terms "chaos stories." Frank states that chaos stories are difficult to listen to or to read, as they have no coherent story structure, timeline, or tick and tock of plot. He contends that chaos stories convey distress and are themselves distressing. They aren't narratives at all. Instead, they are collages, fractured shards of memories, feelings, sensations, and images.

There are times when people have experiences that don't fit neatly into a storyline, a narrative of what happened. Especially within the contexts of trauma, suffering, and oppression, our ability to arrange bits together into a coherent narrative is overwhelmed. Yet these experiences, beyond the reach of narrative, can be formulated, conveyed, and communicated through metaphor, poetry, art, photography, and gesture. Perhaps this is like Virginia Woolf's existential moments of being, moments of knowing, behind the cotton wool of everyday life—moments she conveyed through her "breaking the sequence" style of writing.

Donnel B. Stern, a psychoanalyst and researcher on witnessing, trauma, and dissociation—the defensive splitting of self—contends that there are important nonnarrative ways to organize experiences, as well as times it is best to leave the experiences unorganized. He calls these "the unthought known": experiences that are in some sense known, but are not yet (or perhaps ever) available to reflective thought or verbalization. They are a type of implicit knowing—there but not there. Metaphor, poetry, art, photography, and gesture speak directly to our implicit knowing.

Listen carefully. Here is the chaos illness narrative version of my story, told through the fractured bits and fragments of my life as recorded in my journals and poems:

I have often asked myself the reason for the sadness,
in a world where tears are just a lullaby.
Thump.
The door closes

because it was so old and fragile. So I called it my sick doll. She had no other name. The doll had blue glass eyes that opened and closed, and long wavy blond hair—real hair, my mother told me, a fact I found bizarre. But I was more interested in the contents of the second box.

Before she opened this box, my mother would grow quiet and gaze out of my bedroom window, while absentmindedly caressing my forearm. Then she'd open the box, pull out a leather pouch full of old, musty-smelling letters, a sepia-colored photograph, and a Nazi armband with tiny, even stitches all around the black swastika. She told me the photo was of Jack Murray, her fiancé, an artist who was killed in the Normandy invasion. She let me hold the photograph and the armband, but not the letters.

Jack was tall and handsome, with a wide grin. At those times, I wondered who I would have been if Jack had been my father. Would I even exist?

Of the many mysteries of my childhood and of my parents, this one stands out as among the strangest. My three older siblings insist that my mother never did this with them when they were sick, and that they only knew of the Nazi armband from when she mentioned it offhandedly while they studied World War II in high school. So why me, and why when I was sick? I never asked my mother, as I suspected she wouldn't be able to tell me. When she died in 2008, I inherited the doll, the letters, the photograph, her aquamarine engagement ring from Jack—and the Nazi armband.

Tracing these stories, I realize how intergenerational trauma occurs, how insidious it is, how it seeps into the pores during fevers and open sores. I now see the connection between this deeper illness story and my hallucinated personal narrative. The nonsensical storyline of escaping a Nazi concentration camp that flashed through my head when I had hypothermia. The story that helped me survive the open-water swim. Stories, story fragments, moldering letters, metaphors—they come to us unbidden, and they pull us either under, or through.

In *The Wounded Storyteller*, Arthur Frank states, "To tell one's life is to assume responsibility for that life," and by witnessing to our own stories, we are able to mourn not only for ourselves, but for others. Witness is a relationship. It draws us in as participants. If we listen, if we see, we are witnesses; we are implicated and affected even if we avert our eyes, close our ears, turn our backs.

But to take on this responsibility, we need to expand the possibilities of forms of witnessing, of telling our stories. We also need to find ways to increase our capacity to listen to—and to hear—different types of illness stories, including the more distressing chaos stories.

Feminist literary scholars Susan S. Lanser and Hélène Cixous point out that fractured stories, lyric stories, chaos stories are forms more commonly used by women and marginalized people. Not surprisingly, these forms are themselves marginalized.

Now each word is a poem,
draw knowledge softer,
suckle life from all splinters,
embrace shadows beyond words.

This was part of a poem I wrote on the back of a ferry-crossing fare receipt in the fall of 2014 soon after my father died. At the time, I was simultaneously on a writing retreat on Whidbey Island and teaching community health with a health humanities flare to nursing students in Seattle. During times of intense emotional turmoil, I am tossed out of narrative. I wrote poems while crossing the Puget Sound, back and forth to work and to retreat.

It requires more effort on the part of readers, of listeners, of health care providers to allow people the space and time it takes to tell their illness stories in whichever form they want, including in the more realistic chaos or fractured or broken narrative form. It requires more effort to be able to listen to, to hear, these stories. It requires being able to stay within the cold, gray waters of uncertainty, the waters from which spring life.

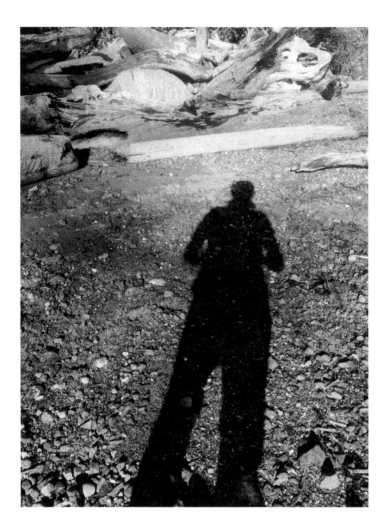

Five

Listen, Carefully

The fact that we are here and that I speak now these words is an attempt to break the silence and bridge some of those differences between us, for it is not difference which immobilizes us, but silence.
—Audre Lorde

<u>Listen, carefully</u>. The whine of a seaplane. The perky ping of email. The crackle of my crumpled-paper thoughts tossed onto the floor.

<u>Listen carefully</u>. I'm sitting in a clinic exam room trying to obtain a coherent medical history from a forty-five-year-old homeless patient. Her pink pants strain over ample thighs, gray sweatshirt dribble-stained, a miasmic aura of tobacco and brew. I listen to her story—or rather to her looping, swirling, spitting, splitting multiplicities of stories—but am distracted by her pinched face, wild-flying hands, charred stubble teeth. She pauses, coughs in my direction. I hand her a tissue and lean back, away, on my exam stool. "What kind of operation did you have on your foot? Which hospital? How long ago?" I need you to answer my questions, succinctly please.

She's a difficult patient. She's a slovenly patient. Slovenly, there in the list of patient descriptors in the electronic medical record system on the screen in front of me. That sounds right. The *Oxford English Dictionary* definition of *slovenly*: dirty, disreputable, loutish, and lewd.

<u>Listen carefully</u>. To our medical words, the terms we use, the terms I use. Difficult patient, as in annoying, angry, afraid, ambivalent, alternative-

medicine-believing, noncompliant, questioning, confused, sad, list-bearing, narcotic-seeking, chronic pain-in-the-ass patient. There's a *Physician's Field Guide to the Difficult Patient Interview*, a chapter for each type.

If you stop to listen, to question the words used, you may never finish this medical encounter. You may not get past the history-taking part. How do you take a history? Chief complaint, history of present illness, past medical history, family medical history, social history, and review of systems—the history of your organs. This is our common language: standardized, logical, neat, no room for chaos. History-taking is stealing, erasing, editing. History-taking is what you hear from the messy illness narrative the patient coughs up. Your job is to select a few words, perhaps a pithy phrase, to place in quotation marks under Chief Complaint, in the Subjective findings, in the patient's own words. *Subjective* belongs to the patient. *Subjective* is suspect, suspicious, specious. *Objective* is me, my words, my physical exam and test findings, my diagnosis, my treatment plan. There is no room for subjective me.

Listen carefully. I only have time for one chief complaint. If you tell me many, I'll choose the one I want to pay attention to, the one I think the simplest to diagnose and treat so I can send you on your way and wash my hands, remove your skin cells, your germs, your odor. At the end of the day I peel my clothes into the washer. Standing in the flow of shower, I remember where the patient coughed, where the touch occurred, where the transfer of mucus, skin cells, bacteria, virions, fungi spores—of words—occurred. I scrub them clean. Only the words remain. Their words, my words, the silent spaces in between.

Listen, carefully. I must remember: there is no room for subjective me. *Do not question what you're doing*, I tell myself. It will only drive you crazy. It will drive you away from this place of work; it will drive you never to return, here, back to the chief complaint, history of present illness, past medical history, family medical history, social history, and review of systems—the history of their organs.

Listen carefully. (Ten seconds of silence.) What did you hear? Did you hear yourself squirm? Did people clear their throats? Did someone cough nearby, and you pondered the history of their present illness? Did you wonder if I've lost my mind, my place?

Listen carefully. To the pregnant pause, uncomfortable silence, wise silence, silent treatment, silent infection, silent prayer—to the poet's silent-speaking words. What to make of silence?

Silence is censure, stricture, repress and suppress. Silence is submissive, resistless, yielding. Silence is looking away; silence is not speaking up.

Silence is space, resistance, stance, stone. Silence is protective, private, present. Silence is power.

Listen carefully. To the patient's illness narrative. Listen first to the patient's description of symptom, duration, location, precipitating events. Listen also for the story, time scaffolding, structure, frame, and diction. Listen for the use of metaphors. *I am as cut off from life as sitting inside a car on a rainy day. There's a shackle on my left foot dragging me down, an ice pick in my eye. The ringing in my ears is like a thousand cicadas have landed on my head in the heat of a summer day. In my despair, Medusa has turned me to stone.*

Are you wowed by words, distracted by diction, tantalized by time, mesmerized by metaphor, just as you ponder precipitating events? Are you blinded by your own bloody brilliance? What have you missed by paying attention?

Listen, carefully. If I told you at the beginning to pay attention to my diction, my metaphors, my use of time, my tone, the structure of this story, how would you listen? Would you hear me?

Listen carefully. To the pinched face, wild-flying hands, charred stubble teeth. To the crackle of crumpled-paper thoughts tossed onto the floor. To the history of our present illness. To a thousand cicadas in the heat of a summer day.

Listen, carefully. What do you hear—here—right now?

Six

Where the Homeless Go

From this day forth
I shall be called a wanderer …
—Basho

At the close of a rare cloudless day in Seattle, I ride my bike down a quiet residential street lined with daffodils and into the darkening ink of the sky. I am headed to a homeless youth shelter in the University District. I teach at the university nearby. Tonight, I'll be helping health science students provide foot care to homeless young people.

I connect with the bike trail leading past the university football stadium under construction. The stadium looms like giant excavator buckets howling at the moon. The area is spotted with orange cranes stilled in the dusk. They are draped with red lights, blinking along with the beacon on the hospital tower across the street. I sneer at the stadium, at its obscene suck of money, at its bulk blocking the view of the pink alpenglow of snowcapped Mount Rainier. I glance over my left shoulder at the darkened concrete wing of the hospital complex where my office is located.

A block before the homeless shelter, I pass a gray-bearded man wearing layers of greasy coats and clutching a stuffed black garbage bag. He is headed towards the gaping mouth of the urban cave across the street: the underground university parking garage where homeless people camp beside steam vents. I watch his slow progress as I push my bike along the cracked sidewalk.

I lock my bike in an alley in the University District, between a pizza place and a scruffy coffee shop. It's a Friday, date night for students, so the places are full of scrubbed young people, laughing and eating. Beside the bike racks, large concrete orbs are artfully arranged and anchored to the pavement. Public art concealing its real aim: to prevent homeless people from sleeping here. I walk past overflowing blue recycling Dumpsters onto a stained loading dock behind a church, and enter the windowless fellowship hall.

in university shadows
homeless wander
paths to refuge

Barefoot

When I was a child, my home was a summer camp in the Virginia countryside. My father was the camp director. I went barefoot all summer, whenever I was out of sight of my father, who had a No Bare Feet policy. With six hundred acres to roam, I was out of my father's sight much of the time. After a day of swimming in the leaf-stained lake, running barefoot through the woods, and playing volleyball on the dirt court in the fields, I'd head home, sneakers tied together and slung over my shoulder.

It was usually fully dark by then, and we were so far from the nearest city that the Milky Way was a dazzling crown above my head. Fireflies flicked upwards at the edge of the woods and bullfrogs recited Tibetan chants from the nearby lake. Walking across the mown grass fields, eddies of moist humus heat lapped across my skin, followed by tendrils of cooler, pine-scented air that made me shiver. The eddies were like spirits playing tag across the grass. My muscles were humming tired; I felt the pull of rest, of climbing into my bed piled with stuffed animals and books. I had memorized the path that cut through the woods from the edge of the field to my house in the oak forest. My toes grasped exposed tree roots and my body swayed to the rhythm of the winding path. Camp fit me like a well-worn pair of shoes.

In the bright lights of our house, my mother stared at my feet, ringed in sediment layers of ochre dust. She frowned and said, "I see you've been running around barefoot again. Go wash those feet before bed!" Then she smiled. Later she came to my bedroom, kissed me good night, and told me not to let the bedbugs bite.

Tonight in the homeless shelter, a nineteen-year-old young man from Georgia says, "My momma always told me not to go barefoot and I didn't listen. That's why my feets so bad. And I have to walk everywhere on 'em now." He reaches down and gently rubs his gnarled brown feet, soaking in a white plastic basin. His feet are darkly scarred and calloused: the feet of an old man.

walking barefoot
we find our way
though cruel paths scar

Lottery

A thin, pimply faced man at the shelter tells me, "People who have ADHD are more ticklish," followed by, "Cancer is excess energy—if you don't use it right, it turns on you." He's probably speaking from experience, so I nod in agreement.

Sitting nearby on a frayed couch is a small young man wearing oversized glasses, looking like a rumpled version of Harry Potter. In a soft, barely audible voice, he tells me he just walked forty miles from his rural home to Seattle, following the railroad tracks. He has a badly twisted ankle from falling on the railbed rocks. I notice his boots have duct tape holding the soles together.

There are close to forty-five homeless young people staying at the shelter tonight. Most nights their names are chosen by a lottery system, because there aren't enough beds. They must be in the shelter by 8:30 p.m. for bed check. As their names are called, they are handed a blue plastic tub containing clean sheets and are assigned a numbered mat on the floor. The thick mats are covered with blue tarp material, because bedbugs happen to be real. Most of the young people have sleeping mats on the floor; a lucky few get to sleep on one of several bunk beds located on the perimeter. The bunk beds afford more privacy and the semblance of home. From the corner of my eye I notice a young woman curled up in a bottom bunk, headphones on. She is clutching a well-worn stuffed animal and writing in her journal.

young outcasts cluster
numbered pallets on the floor
what do they tell us?

Journey

The homeless young people sleep under maps. One long wall of the fellow-ship hall is covered with maps of all the states and territories of the United States. A local artist designed the mural as a way to take the edge off the windowless church basement room. She brought in stacks of old maps and had the young people pick one they identified with and decorate it with their stories and drawings. Their maps are outlined in thick blue ink. Combined with other maps, they are arranged in a rough geographical outline of our country. Scattered across the mural, the artist added drawings of her own: anatomical human hearts and sheets of raindrops. A large pair of faceless human eyes and a flock of black crows midflight adorn the top of the mural. I happen to like crows, but the fact they eat their own ill or injured doesn't make them an appealing addition to the shelter.

I am drawn to the words of the young people. The map of Seattle has multiple stories written on it, including "I live here, I play here, skate here, sleep here, date here, work here until next year." California has "So many hot girls live here." A young woman had a two-year prostitution sentence in Myrtle Beach, South Carolina, but thinks, "I hold this city down hella in fact." I have no idea what holding a city down means in this context: Respect? Love? Hate? A young man from Washington, DC, was in foster care and then was adopted. He adds, "I used to have a morbid feeling looking up at the Washington Monument." On the map of Virginia, over my childhood home, there is a drawing of a large empty bed.

maps of belonging
recorded on church walls
yearning to be home

Riding my bike home that night along the dark trail, I remember Basho: "Each day is a journey, the journey itself home."

Seven

Steps to Foot Care

It is appropriate that I sing
The song of the feet
The weight of the body
And what the body chooses to bear
Fall on me
—Nikki Giovanni

* <u>Gloves are not necessary unless skin integrity is impaired</u>.

"No one touches me like that—gently, as if they cared. You know all that crap about good touch and bad touch, like they teach little kids in school nowadays? They don't teach 'em how sometimes you really can't tell the damn difference—pardon my French. Only touch I get these days is from greasy, greedy, fat-fisted fingers groping my body, like I'm a tissue or something they blow their noses in and toss away. Oh shoot! I can tell you don't want to know this stuff about me. I can tell you're all shocked and like you don't know what to say. Don't worry, you don't have to say nothin'.

Please don't change your mind and feel like you gotta put gloves on after all. I like you touching me with no gloves on and not looking all scared about it. Thank you for being down here at the women's shelter this morning, doing this foot care stuff. Ya'll bein' down here volunteering to do this is a blessin'. I can tell you'll make a great doctor or nurse or whatever it is you're studyin' to be. Thank you for not wearing gloves, for being willing to touch me like I'm a real person."

1. <u>Soak bare feet in soothing bath treatment with warm water</u>.

"Put my feet in this here dishpan on the floor? OK, but that's the same kinda dishpan I used to wash my dishes in back when I had my own apartment. Let's see, how long ago was that? God, I don't even remember now. That apartment sucked! The sink was so nasty and overrun with cockroaches I had to use a dishpan like this one here I could keep halfway clean. Now I miss that apartment. At least it wasn't this crazy-ass shelter full of drama queens and all their fights. You wouldn't believe some of the things that happen down here! The staff—they try to keep the real nut cases outta here, but there's some nasty catfights with some of these women hittin' an screamin' an scratchin'. They call each other "slut" or "loser"—you know, bad names like that—then it'll just start an all-out war. I stay out of it as much I can—keep to myself and don't take no sides in all them fights, cause if I do, then I'm likely to get myself hit upside the head when I'm not lookin'. Ain't worth it, I tell ya that much. I can't wait to get outta here!

It feels sort of odd seeing my feet in that there dishpan. They look kinda sad sittin' there in that water, don't they? I guess I don't pay enough attention to my feet—they look all gnarly and wore out. I remember my momma had this cheap ole foot massager thing. She'd sit in a big ole easy chair in the livin' room in the trailer we lived in. She'd kick off her clunky work shoes, light up a cigarette, and put her feet in that machine, and just lay back and sigh real hard. She worked herself to death, that's what I think. I get sad when I think of Momma. She did a lot of waitressin' at the truck stop diner near where we lived. She's mostly the one fed us kids, cause Daddie? He worked in this pine mill but he didn't always have no steady work, and he really didn't have no steady work when he started drinkin' hard. You can't be drinkin' and operatin' them big ole saws. He got to be missin' some of his fingers that way, but it didn't stop his drinkin'. He had enough fingers to keep a hold that glass of whisky!

I guess you guys sterilize these pans or something between people, right? Some of these women here don't keep themselves clean, and I wouldn't want to catch their cooties. Oooo-eee! No way I want no cooties! Just like in grade school, we used to say Johnnie or whatnot, he's got the cooties and run away? We thought it was real funny, but then the cooties got real and it weren't so funny no more."

2. <u>Use soap to wash feet, then remove soap with water.</u>

"That soap you're usin' there, that oatmeal stuff? I remember my momma usin' it on me when I had the chicken pox real bad and was scratchin' myself to death. Them white pockmark scars there on my leg is where they got all infected from me scratchin' 'em raw. I thought them chicken pox sores was the cooties for sure, cause they said I caught 'em from some kid at school. I was a little bitty thing an didn't like takin' no baths. But Momma? She said that stuff the doctor told her was like medicine and it was real expensive so it had better work, and I'd sure as hell better get my butt in that bathtub! It did make me feel better while I was in that tub, but once I was out I started scratchin' all over again. I was too little to know that soap wasn't magic like my momma said. It smells real good though, don't it now?"

3. <u>Dry feet, especially in between toes.</u>

"That blue hospital towel thing you're using to dry my feet—they're the same kinds a ones they use at the clinic where I go get checked out. Lie down on that doctor's table, put my feet up in those nasty metal clamps. They put those same blue towels under my butt. I hate those exams. They ask me all these real personal questions, and it don't seem none of their business. They teach you all in school to ask them types a questions? Them clinic doctors and nurses look at me all different like when I tell 'em I don't really have no husband or boyfriend or nothin'. Then they ask me—or they wants to ask me—Then how come you got this STD thing or this pregnancy we be checking you for? You sure as hell don't get it from no toilet seat! As if I'm a retard. It's bad out here in Seattle cause a my accent. They think I gotta be stupid cause I talk all country-like. They never knew a smart person from the country? I may have a country accent and I may not have finished school, but I ain't dumb. You can't be dumb and survive them streets out there. No book-learnin' helps you on those streets, I tell you that much.

Oh yeah. I was tellin' ya bout that pelvic exam thing. Somethin' weird always happens to me during those exams, and I've always wondered if it happens to other women or if I got somethin' wrong inside my head. When my feet's up in the air like that and the doctor's got that dang plastic thing up inside me poking around like a jackhammer? I just go some other place, like I leave my body there on the table for them to do whatever they need to, but I myself—I skedaddle right on outta there. You remember that machine they got on that Star Trek TV show? That one beams you up somewhere, like to a different planet or something? "Beam me up, Scotty!" I remember that. It's just like what happens to me on that there exam table. I beam myself up to some nice Hawaiian beach like them pictures I seen, but sometimes I just go blank, like I don't know where I end up but maybe inside some dark closet somewheres. Like that beam-me-up machine gets broke and I'm lost in space or in that closet or something. Just when I figure I'm lost forever, then I feel the doctor like pattin' me real hard on my knee and tellin' me he's done now so I can sit up careful like so I don't fall off the table. Well, anyway, that's what them blue hospital towels remind me of. You ever heard anything like that? Like I said, I was always scared to tell anyone that story in case it means I'm a nutcase.

You really want to do this kinda stuff the rest a your life? Yeah, maybe it pays real well, but you can't pay me enough to work at no hospital or clinic or whatnot. Creepy places, I think. I can tell though that you'll be nicer to people than a lot of the doctors and nurses I've had up in my face judgin' me, tellin' me what to do with my life, askin' me how come I got this STD. Ain't none of their business tellin' me what to do or how to live my life! They's supposed to just fix me up, like fix what's broken. They wouldn't like it if someone did that to them, so why's it okay for them to do it to me? That's what I wanna know. They teach you all this in school? I hope they teaches you all some manners with patients, like how to treat patients as if they's your own momma or sisters or whatnot—treat 'em with respect. They should remember they's definitely likely to get old and die some day, and then how they wants to be treated themselves? With some respect, that's right. People like me might be dirt poor and might a not had much schoolin' and had some bad stuff happen to 'em or maybe even done some bad stuff them own selves, but that don't give no one—specially not no doctor or nurse—the right to look down on a person and not treat 'em with respect. We's all human with the same heart. Like the Bible says somewheres or nother: God made us all. No matter what your religion, or even if you ain't got no religion, I don't care: we's all the same."

4. Inspect feet for cuts, blisters, redness, swelling, calluses, etc.

"That there scar? That one's from a dog bite I got back when I was a kid and we was livin' in that trailer park. We was livin' down South, way down right along the Georgia line kinda near Valdosta—ever heard of it? Don't matter. Little bitty town. One part of our trailer was in Georgia; other part was in Florida. Strangest thing to think there's some line you can't see right down the middle of where you livin'. I used to lie in my bunk bed at night and think of it split in two, with me along with it like Houdini or something. Momma told me stop thinkin' such silly thoughts and go on to sleep.

Anyways, that scar. A neighbor had a big ole mean-ass dog that got loose off a his chain and took a chomp outta my foot as I was runnin' past. My daddy, he seen it and come runnin' and kicked that dog real hard fore it could eat me up. Daddy was always wearing them hard cowboy boots with them pointy toes? Dog went a flyin' and a yelpin'! Daddy, he said he wanted to shoot that damn dog, he was so mad. But he was too drunk to know where he left his gun. Would a been funny if I weren't bleeding all over the place. I knew where his gun was, but I didn't want him shootin' that dog—least not right then. My foot hurt too much.

Momma, she borrowed a neighbor's car and took me to the hospital. Those doctors and nurses, they held me down and gave me a ton a stitches and I was screamin' the whole time. I don't think they gave me any numbin' stuff, but maybe they did and it just didn't took right or somethin'. I remember they was talkin' about having to give me a bunch a shots in my tummy in case that dog had rabies. Not sure what happened but I didn't have to get no stomach shots and I didn't start foamin' at the mouth or nothin'. I'm scared to death a dogs now. I cross the street if I sees one comin'."

5. Assess pedal pulses (dorsalis pedis and posterior tibial).

"Oh Lord! That feels sorta weird there what ya doin'! Cause I can feel my heart beatin' there on the inside a my foot when ya presses your fingers on it. Makes me nervous, like you's reachin' in an touchin' my heart in some sorta way.

I remember seein' them nurses do that to my momma's neck when she was dyin'. Cancer got her real young. Like I said, she worked herself to death, that's what she did. And Daddie? He let her do it. I ain't never forgive him for that. Now it's too late and he's dead, too. Not sure I'd ever forgive him though, no matter how long he lived. I know the Bible says we needs to forgive people but I don't see no way no how to do it sometimes.

I was thirteen when my momma died, and that's when my life really went to hell in a handbasket, cause my daddie started drinking even worse after momma died. I guess he really loved her. I had to leave school and earn money any ole way I could. Daddie didn't seem to care. That's when I got in this here mess. I started workin' the truck stop, but not like momma did cause I wasn't old enough to work at no diner. I think if my momma had a lived I wouldn't have gone down this here road—ended up in the life and in this shelter. I thank the Lord I don't have no kids to drag into this shelter with me. I love kids and all, and there's some sweet ones here, but this ain't no place to try and raise 'em, I don't think. And a lot of women here's had their kids taken away by that CPS and those kids end up all abused in foster care like you hear about. That's sad: kids growin' up without their real mommas. I know what that's like. Ain't no kid should a have that happen to 'em.

The trailer park I grew up in wasn't a whole lot better than this shelter from the looks of it, but at least we had our own privacy, and some of our neighbors was like family. Not that guy with the mean-ass dog I told you about. He was a nutcase and people stayed away from him. Most a the others were real good folk. Dirt poor, but all a us was dirt poor together so we kinda took care of each other and no one looked down on ya. Different than in the big city, like here in Seattle, where people mostly keeps to themselves, minds their own business, and don't really help their neighbors like they do in the country. In the South where I'm from, people's friendlier. They looks you in the eye and says hello every time. People here don't do that, I notice. In this here shelter, people come an go so fast you really don't get no time to get to know 'em. And you gotta keep a watch out all the time cause people steals your stuff here. Some a the staff people are real nice, and they do try to make it like a home, but no way—it's no home.

Better than on the streets though, I can tell you that much. For sure. Streets ain't no place for no one but specially not for no woman. Been there and ain't goin' back if I can help it. Got beat up and worse so many times out there on the street, for sure God watchin' over me or I'd long ago be dead—or crazy. I'm on a wait list now to get me an apartment of my own, some sort of transitional place I think they calls it. I seen 'em and they're a whole lot better than this here shelter.

Tryin' to get myself a real job, not what I been doing all these years. Havin' a record with the law don't make it so easy. But I got me a real nice caseworker now—Heidi—you know her? She's sure been a blessin' in my life. She keeps being all positive and makes me feel better about myself and like I can do this, I can have a different life. She even helped me get new clothes for job interviews. New shoes even, cause all my shoes were all high-heeled slutty-like. Feels weird to walk around now in these flat shoes. They make real cute ones now though—not ole-lady ones. Nothin' against ole ladies, mind ya, but I'm not there yet. I want to be an ole lady with style! An ole lady who still takes care of herself, you know what I mean? My nanna now, my momma's momma, she had style! Kinda crazy but not loony-toons crazy. She'd wear these big ole hats with fake flowers all over 'em and wear these long white cotton gloves and bright flowered dresses like she was goin' to a church meetin' all the time. She liked wearing orange, too—said orange was a happy color and she couldn't be sad wearin' that orange."

6. <u>Assess pedal sensation using monofilament</u>.

"Damn! Is that a needle? I don't like no needles anywhere near me! I had a boyfriend once, he was a junkie and he tried to get me hooked on that crap, but I told him no way, I wasn't messin' with no dope or no needles. He dumped me over that. Got hisself another girlfriend who was a junkie. He ended up gettin' hisself AIDS and all—real cooties. He shriveled up and died real fast. Don't know what happened to his girlfriend. She probably got that AIDS disease and died, too. God's been a watchin' out for me that a way, cause doctors say I ain't got the AIDS virus, an I sure wanna keep it that way.

Oh, okay, I see it ain't no needle but some plastic bendy thing. Yeah, you can do your tests with it. Close my eyes? What for? I don't like closin' my eyes; I like keepin' a watch on things. Only way to stay safe in this world. Gets in the way a sleepin' sometimes though. I don't want to close my eyes and not know what's happenin' round me. If I don't have my own room I can lock the bedroom door on, I don't sleep real good. Kinda stay up with my eyes open, pinchin' myself to stay awake until after a while I just sorta pass out I guess. Almost like when I was little and stayed awake worrying I'd be split in two sleepin' right there on that state line. But I got worse things on my mind nowadays. That's why I really wants that apartment soon, so I can get me some sleep. Sleep's gotta be one of the most important things for your health, don't ya think? Not just beauty sleep but sanity sleep, that's what I call it: sanity sleep. I always feel better about myself and the world when I get me some good sleep. I stay away from sleepin' pills though. Them things is dangerous. I know people almost killed themselves with them pills.

Yeah, I feel that. You pokin' me on the bottom of my foot with that needle-lookin' thing. Tickles. I'm real ticklish. Some guys they use that against me, like a distraction or diversion or whatnot. Kinda paralyzes me so they can do something with me I don't wanna do. Oh, never mind all that stuff. You look like you're a nice clean young lady who don't let no guys do bad things to you. You stay that way now, ya hear?"

7. <u>Cut nails straight across with clippers.</u>

"Nah, I'll do that myself. Ain't no one cut my nails the way I like 'em cut. Wish I had me some nail polish, I'd polish 'em now. They look all nasty with the polish chipped off. Some guys, they have themselves some foot fetish for sure! Won't have nothin' to do with a woman unless she has nice feet with nail polish and nice shoes and all. Crazy, right? Like who really cares what someone's feet looks like! But I do like keepin' myself clean and lookin' as pretty as I can all over. Makes me feel better bout myself. So even if no one looks at my feet 'cept me, I like to keep 'em nice. Specially now with nice weather comin' long and I can wear sandals again, I gotta get me some nail polish. I gotta girlfriend here I can borrow some from. They gots some real strange nail colors now, like green and black and stuff? I leave that to the youngsters; ain't for me. I only use red or pink on my nails. More classic-like."

8. <u>Smooth off sharp edges with emery board.</u>

"I'll do that myself, too, after I cut 'em. Can't stand it when there's a rough spot gets stuck on my stockings and ruins 'em. Those things get expensive, but I don't feel real dressed unless I got me some stockings on. Even when it's hot, I gotta have them stockings on. Is how my momma raised me, even though she wouldn't let me wear no stockings until I was sixteen, and she died afore that anyway. My nanna—my momma's momma like I said, the one wore orange? She wore stockings all the time. She died fore momma did or I'd a gone and lived with her after momma was gone. She would a raised me right and not turned me loose like my daddie, he did."

9. <u>Gently remove calluses and dead skin with pumice stone</u>.

"Oh yeah, I got me some mean ole nasty hard spots on my feet, specially those back there on my heels. See 'em right there? Don't know why, but some of my shoes just rubs 'em the wrong way or somethin'. Starts off a hurting and after a while I can't feel nothin' there. Just like some things in life, right? Like a broken heart or something. Haaah! Starts off a hurtin' like hell and then just goes numb till maybe the next one comes along and starts hurtin' all over again. Wish I could rub away the piled-up hurt places inside me like I can those callous places on my feet. Wouldn't that be something if they invented a way to do that? Ain't sure no one but Jesus can do that kinda thing though.

I think a heaven sometimes: like the preacher, he says in heaven ain't gonna be no more hurtin' and wailin'? Makes me real sad what I've done in my life, and I sure wanna get to heaven. But you know, Jesus, he even saved bad people like prostitutes and lepers and whatnot, so I guess I can be saved, too. I keep on prayin' on it."

10. <u>Gently remove any debris around nails with wooden stick</u>.

"Oooh yuck! That toe gunk stinks! You make sure you wash your hands real well so you don't go outta here smellin' like no toe gunk. Smells like somethin' died in there and gone all rotten and decomposin'.

Used to have roadkill, like dogs or deer got themselves killed along the country road we lived on, and in summer that hot sun would beat on 'em. They'd get all swole up and bust and smell for miles round! Oooo-eee! Nasty big ole black flies all over 'em, and turkey buzzards, they'd finally come along and pick 'em clean down to the bones. I used to have to walk along that road and hitchhike places and I hated that smell. Sometimes it'd be so bad I'd pick some wild roses and honeysuckle from side a the road and just keep 'em up near my nose to get me through till the air cleared.

You got yourself a boyfriend? He treat you real nice and buys you flowers and stuff? I love flowers. I buy 'em for myself whenever I can. Your boyfriend don't never hit you now, does he? I don't stand for none of them hittin' men. They slap me or push me just one time an I'm outta there, don't never go back for no more. I got girlfriends though—some of 'em here in this shelter with me—they seem smart and all but they can't seem to stay away from them hittin'-type a men. They like 'em for some reason. I don't get it. But then, the stuff I've let guys do to me, I guess it's all the same, or maybe what I do is even worse, I don't know. Makes me all sad to think about it, but it's been creeping back into my head more lately. Maybe cause I'm away from that life right now I can see it more? Or maybe cause Heidi, she pushes me to think about it and she tells me it's time to be good to myself and not beat myself up over things I couldn't do nothin' about. Things from when I was a real little girl I never told no one bout till Heidi come along.

Not sure why I trusts her so much. She's seen me through some real bad times and she's hung in there with me. But she's having a baby now and she just told me she's gotta leave soon to care for that little baby—that she's not gonna do this work no more, leastwise not for a while. That'll be the luckiest baby alive with her as its momma!

She trying to get me to start seein' some other caseworker, but I don't want to start all over again spillin' my guts out and all with a stranger. I'd rather not have no caseworker if I can't have Heidi, but she says that's bullshit, if you'll pardon my words there, but that's just what she said. Straight up: that's bullshit! I like that about her—she don't pussyfoot around, she just comes right out and tells me what she's thinking, all honest-like. I reckon she's got a point though. I gotta learn to trust some people if I'm gonna get outta this mess I'm in. That's another thing I pray about: findin' me some trust and knowin' who I can trust, who won't screw me over. Just like that good touch, bad touch thing: it's hard to tell the difference, but I guess there's a way to figure it out."

11. <u>Apply lotion to feet, but NOT between toes.</u>

"Oooh! That feels so good! I could sit here all day an let you do that—no really, I could! It's like bein' at a spa or somethin'—feels all pamperin'-like. Thanks so much for this whole foot thing. It kinda makes me feel better all over. When your feet feel good you can't help but feel good. Strangest thing now, don't ya think? They teach you in school some reason why that's so? Somethin' in the nervous system, like maybe nerves in the feet's attached to the feel-good center in our heads or something?

They oughta study that more, like they study everything else under the sun. Study somethin' useful like that cause then maybe people wouldn't get so sick all the time or all angry and hurtin' each other. Maybe they wouldn't have to take no feel-good drugs no more. I don't know, sounds like a crazy idea maybe, but keep it in mind when you's out there treatin' people.

You stay sweet and take care a yourself. I be seein' ya round maybe or—no, I take that back—no offense, but I hope I don't see ya, cause like I say, I'm hoping to be outta here soon, get my own apartment and get myself a real job. Anyways, thanks for doing this whole foot thing today. Makes me have hope we gonna have us some better doctors and nurses out there practicin' soon. That sure is a good thing. God bless you; you take care now, ya hear?"

Eight

Foot Notes

How many times these low feet staggered—
—Emily Dickinson

1. <u>Footprints are witness to our beginnings and proof of our existence</u>. I have my son's footprints from when he was a few hours old. I helped hold him still in order to get a set of prints to place in his baby book. Strong-willed and squirmy from the start, Jonathan's right footprint has ten smeary toes. There's a large Y etched in the skin of his right heel.

2. <u>Footprints are witness to our uniqueness, to our individuality</u>. Not even identical twins have the same foot- and handprints, because the prints are a combination of genetic and environmental factors. The infant palm and sole carry traces of the in utero landscape: changes in blood flow, in the alchemy of the placenta, and in the composition of oceanic amniotic fluid. What affects the mother affects the developing fetal body, including the ancient hieroglyphs written on its soles and palms. The unique identifying patterns—the ridges and whorls—in foot- and handprints develop by the twelfth week of fetal life. Once the prints are set, they can be altered only if the deepest layer of skin is damaged.

3. <u>Footprints testify to what we are given and to what we make of what we are given</u>. My son's left newborn footprint is much clearer than his right. In newborns, the skin is thickest on the ball of the foot—the friction ridge at the base of the big toe. It's these identifying "ball prints" in babies that are best. Now that I know to look there, I see that infant Jonathan has two prominent parallel lines, like a musical score, across this ridge, and an arch in the shape of a normal distribution bell curve or a portion of a sine wave

charted through it. Perhaps Jonathan was meant to be musical, or to have an affinity for physics, for statistics, for normality. Adult Jonathan is a historian asking questions of the past.

4. The scientific study of foot- and handprints is dermatoglyphics: skin carvings. The official terms for the identifying patterns in foot- and handprints include *minutia, island, fork, lake, comb, end, fibular loops, open fields, tented loops, double spiral whirls, concentric whorls, distal loops, nascent ridges,* and *triarii*—the heavy infantry of the Roman Army.

5. Footprints can go missing. I have my mother's baby book from her birth in 1923. It somehow survived the Great Kanto Earthquake, tsunami, and firestorms in Japan, where she was born to American missionary parents. Her official birth certificate was destroyed in the Tokyo dragon twist fire. In her baby book, there's a page designated for hand- and footprints, but in their place is a small rice paper package with "Baby's nail clippings—five days old" written across it and a wisp of fine baby hair tied with a bow of pink silk ribbon. The baby hair and wings of ribbon look like a delicate dragonfly.

6. Foot- and handprints are found only in primates; as unique identifiers, they are not otherwise found in nature. The closest are the whorls in the bark of some trees, or the patterned layers of calcification in inner ear stones of vertebrates. The raised ridges and whorls of our foot- and handprints seem to exist for feeling and gripping. They enable touch to be more sensitive to the texture of objects, and they improve gripping—of tree branches for climbing and of tools for fighting and foraging. Our palms and soles have the densest concentration of nerve endings in the body. The soles of our feet are highly sensory because they tell us where we are in relation to the earth. Many Native American tribes consider feet sacred because they have the most direct contact with the earth; barefoot is believed to be the best way to connect with Earth's energy.

7. Neolithic cave artwork includes hand- and footprint designs. Mummies over two thousand years old have ridge patterns on palms and soles that are clearly discernable.

8. Foot- and handprints foretell fortunes. Did our ancestors sit around fires at night gazing at the lines and swirls in each other's hands and feet, prophesying what they meant? Were they closer to the meanings of the hieroglyphs etched in the skin? Now, the patterns and proposed meanings

are available on the internet, so people can examine their palms and soles, searching for answers to their questions: How long will I live? Will I be prosperous or poor? Will I be lucky in love? How many children will I have? Am I headstrong and intense or laid-back and mellow?

9. Footprints are used in medicine and public health. The Gates Foundation has funded an Australian global health project called Happy Feet. The researchers studied the feasibility of using infant footprints as accurate, low-cost biomarkers for tracking childhood vaccination programs in low-resource countries.

10. Footprints record where we've been; footprints follow us more surely than our shadows.

11. Footprints and shoe prints are used by forensic scientists to track the movements of victims and suspects of crimes. Every morning at an intersection near my home, I walk on a section of pavement imprinted with lug-soled boots, which appear to be a men's size ten. The footprints are headed towards an opening in a fence around an empty lot with a moss-covered shed in the far corner. Did a homeless person seek shelter here late one night, cutting across a patch of wet pavement?

12. The soles of our feet carry traces of everywhere we've been. I massaged my mother's feet as she lay dying in a hospice bed. Most touch caused her pain, since she was dying of cancer and stoically refused pain medication—until I began to slip the bright-pink liquid morphine into her milk. But she loved for me to massage her feet, and she asked for it over and over as she lost consciousness and was carried into her dark night.

13. Feet take us to new territory; they witness and record our journey.

Nine

Way Out; Way Home

Home? The edge of the alphabet where words crumble and all form of communication between the living are useless. One day we who live at the edge of the alphabet will find our speech.
—Janet Frame

First, a brief review of one of those ancient Greek myths you've probably heard about but don't remember in detail. Ariadne was the daughter of King Minos of Crete. Her free-spirit forest- and sea-loving mother, Pasiphae, mated with an exotic white bull from the sea and gave birth to Ariadne's half-brother the Minotaur, who was also half-human, half-bull.

The Minotaur, being a bull in a china shop, so to speak, and prone to rages and the eating of maidens and young men, was contained at the center of a labyrinth built by the ingenious inventor Daedalus. Daedalus, like a doting uncle, had made hanging marionette dolls for young Ariadne, and had given her a magic ball of thread. Some versions of the myth call the thread flaxen, or gold, and others say it was life-blood red. When Ariadne fell in love with Prince Theseus, who was intent on slaying the Minotaur, she agreed to help him if he would marry her and take her away to his hometown of Athens. Using her magic ball of thread—the end of which Ariadne tied to the door of the labyrinth—Theseus killed the Minotaur and emerged again triumphant. He married Ariadne and sailed off with her towards Athens, but abandoned her—sleeping—on the island of Naxos, where—once awakened—she promptly married the much more fun-loving Dionysus—god of wine and protector of the homeless.

Now, I want to tell you a story. About stories. About words. About how they guide and pull us through the torn, the thorny places of our lives. About how they falter. About how they reconnect us—to ourselves and to each other.

Ariadne stands guard. Tether yourself to her red thread. Tie the end to the threshold—there—the threshold you stepped over on your way here. Never mind the body lying inert in the doorway. It takes a while to get used to stepping over bodies. The body is there to remind you of those who went before, of those who tried to find their way out, their way home.

1.

Choose carefully which path to take.

Tread lightly between the trees. Trust your instincts. Relax and feel the fir needles beneath your feet. Follow the narrow forest path where the white-tailed deer walk quietly in single file.

> *Hold the silence*
> *like sunbeams through branches*
> *spun in gilded cocoons*
> *rain down*
> *softly, reverently.*

> *Hold the silence*
> *as you enter here.*
> *This is no solitary path*
> *where you pass yourself*
> *going the other way.*

2.

Remember where you came from? The dirt you first stuffed into your gummy mouth? The dirt you toddled over on your way to words? The red thread a ribbon in your hair, the laces on your soft-soled shoes?

> *Shadowed self*
> *beneath blood moon,*
> *hoot owl calls through thickets*
> *of scarlet poison-ivy—*
> *tendrils caress*
> *silver-grayed drifts of time.*

3.

Close your eyes for a moment. What is your earliest memory? It holds the key to who you are, and to where you are headed.

Feathered breath
pressed in parchment.
Chewed mulberry leaves
feed worms that spit
filaments of fiber.

4.

Consider the beauty. There must have been something beautiful, no matter how fleeting. Something to hold on to. Consider the beauty.

Prepare to drift in free fall
through fractured sky.
Bones stripped bare
turned to alphabet runes.

5.

The passageway darkens. The plot thickens. There may be turbulence ahead. In the event of an emergency, oxygen masks will fall down, appearing like dancing marionettes. Secure yours over your mouth and nose before helping others. Prepare yourself. You could lose your way.

Going under,
shunt through searing halls
on your way to surgery
to correct the stutter
to loosen the sibilant tongue
to extract the chimera
of what is you and not you.

6.

Although you have yet to reach the center of the labyrinth, arguably the climax of this story, you begin to feel the presence of the Minotaur, smell the fetid breath. With its centrifugal force, you are pulled inextricably deeper.

There is no refuge here.

Bats sing call and response
hymns through ink-dust skies.

Default normals used
in place of guardian spirits
trailing
torn bandages of words
wound in fern-frond fists.

7.

Congratulations! You made it through that difficult patch. I see you doubled back and tied yourself in a knot. And your heart skipped a beat from the looks of that EKG strip. The phosphorus I was able to extract from your blood now illuminates your path—although first you must remove the gauze covering your eyes, spit the cotton from your mouth, and learn to speak again. Raise your right index finger if you can hear me, if you understand.

Stained silk stigmata
stored through lines of women
in mothballed cedar chests
as if a treasure.

8.

Caution. This is where it gets interesting. This is the center. Slay the Minotaur. It's up to you to decide how to do that.

Gaze into the face of the abyss.
Chaos is a game played with spiraled doodles
that spell nothingness.

Trace fingerprints to their source,
etched lines ricochet
and echo through the night.

Gather shredded selves
stitched lovingly
with mosaic thread.

9.

It's tempting to run back out into the world, to scream, "I killed the monster! I survived to tell the tale! I win the prize! Ariadne, I'm taking you to a Greek island for an all-expense paid vacation!" But in your excitement, you forget that your odyssey is not over. And you forget that Ariadne is not the prize. She belongs to no one.

There is no resilience here,
Bounce back, bend, return to steady state.

The body remembers
there is no resilience here.
But there is resistance, stance, stories
and scars of our sick-sweet journey.

10.

See, I warned you. You were so excited about reaching the center of the labyrinth, of slaying that stinking hybrid, of thinking that was your goal, that you dropped the ball of red thread. You now face a dead end, blind alley, end of the road—a different sort of resistance: you have hit the proverbial ...

Hieroglyphic wall; no way out.
Retrace your steps to the last glint of light;
follow it forward through blue emptiness.

11.

All this mystic blue. Maggie Nelson writes that blue is "something of an ecstatic accident produced by void and fire." Goethe claims we love blue "because it draws us after it."

Pause there
while the sea lights a candle
and stringed surf
washes you clean.

12.

Assemble the strands together—words, images, gestures, metaphors. They are all equally important mementos. Pack them in a satchel and prepare to

...

Spin the way home.
And look back
to a time …

When words were poems,
our body's understanding
was written in flesh;
a repose, a prayer whispered
in answer to awe.
Round marbled babbles sang praise,
danced the sun on waves.

Now each word is a poem,
draw knowledge softer,
suckle life from all splinters,
embrace shadows beyond words.

Hold the silence
as you exit there.
Quiet pandemonium
calls you home.

Gaze into that mirror—
Listen, as Eduardo Galeano whispers in your ear:
Mirrors are filled with people.
The invisible see us.
The forgotten recall us.
When we see ourselves, we see them.
When we turn away, do they?

Gaze into this mirror—
Listen, as I whisper in your ear:
Home is where you are known.
You are not alone.
The key is tied
to the way out and the way home.

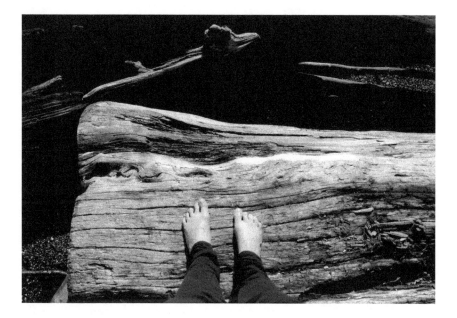

Ten

Past Forgiveness

Forgetting is something that time alone takes care of, but forgiveness is an act of volition, and only the sufferer is qualified to make the decision.
—Simon Wiesenthal

In *Regarding the Pain of Others*, Susan Sontag writes of the meaning of images depicting tragedies and traumas. Towards the end of the book she contends, "There is simply too much injustice in the world. And too much remembering (of ancient grievances: Serbs, Irish) embitters. To make peace is to forget. To reconcile, it is necessary that memory be faulty and limited."

But I wonder if reconciling, if forgiving, is always predicated on forgetting. And, is forgiving always a good thing?

As I began writing this essay, a young white supremacist shot and killed nine black people during a prayer service in a historic black church in Charleston, South Carolina. The day after this hate crime atrocity, the relatives of those murdered came together and gave a public declaration in which they called on the shooter to confess his crime and repent. He was not admitting to any wrongdoing or crime, yet they forgave him for murdering their loved ones. They said that they called on their deeply held Christian convictions to guide them in this matter.

Was their quick and very public forgiveness a form of Christian witnessing, a rebuke to the devil, to evil in the world? Or was it something else? I realize I am treading on difficult ground here, that being within my white privilege, I can never know what the family members of those victims experienced. Of course, there is something admirable and noble in turning anger and vengeance into love and forgiveness. But then that becomes the standard, and what if there are relatives of victims who can't or do not want to forgive the white supremacist murderer?

Forgiveness is a peculiarly Christian thing to do. Having been raised within an exclusively Christian worldview—with its *turn the other cheek, forgive a person seventy times seven, forgive us our debts as we forgive our debtors*—I hadn't realized that other major world religions have different views on forgiveness. In Judaism, forgiveness can only be granted by the aggrieved person, and only after the perpetrator has asked for forgiveness and has made both atonement and restitution.

Forgiveness is also a peculiarly female thing to do; it is emphasized in traditional gender roles in Eastern and Western societies. Women are conditioned to be the family and community peacemakers, and forgiving is viewed as an essential part of that role. People who forgive are supposed to soften their hearts and release their anger and sense of revenge in nonviolent, nonliteral ways.

Robert D. Enright, a Catholic psychologist at the University of Wisconsin–Madison, has developed a sixty-item forgiveness inventory to measure forgiveness, and an eight-step program leading to forgiveness. He has been dubbed "Dr. Forgiveness." Through his research, he contends that people who forgive lead healthier and longer lives than those who "stay stuck" or "hold on to" resentment and lack of forgiveness. He advocates using the "two-chair technique" when counseling someone to forgive. The person seeking to forgive sits in one chair and faces an empty chair representing the person who wronged them. They tell that person—that chair—how they feel. Then they sit in the second chair and try to see things from the other person's perspective. They talk things through with the imaginary person until they achieve forgiveness.

There is even an International Forgiveness Day, the first Sunday of August, established by the World Wide Forgiveness Alliance. The 2015 International Forgiveness Day was on August 2, and at 2:00 p.m. on that day, people were called "to take two minutes to forgive someone and join over two million people in the Wave of Forgiveness." The website features photographs and testimonials of the 2015 Heroes and Champions of Forgiveness. Most were women, and it seems that most were women of color—a fact I find ironic given the power dynamics inherent in forgiveness. I took a thirty-three-item online forgiveness quiz that included questions such as "Forgiveness is a sign of weakness" and "I believe that revenge is devilish and forgiveness is saintly"—an echo of Alexander Pope's famous line of poetry "To err is human; to forgive, divine."

The quiz questions used a Likert scale, and most of my answers were neutral because my real answer to these questions was "It depends." Nevertheless, my composite score told me I tended to be a more forgiving person. Even though I thought it a rather silly and oversimplified test—and I question our society's insistence on forgiveness, especially gendered forgiveness—I find my test result to be comforting. I also find that comfort disquieting.

I have spent my entire life—or at least my entire life from when I first became fully aware of myself—trying to find a way to forgive my dysfunctional family. Mainly my father, the charismatic narcissist minister who liked to grope my budding breasts and then pretend he had only been trying to show me fatherly affection. Or that he was only sponging my chest, when I was ill in bed with a high fever from red measles when I was fourteen. "What kind of Freudian psychological hang-ups do you have about your father?" he asked, when I grew old enough to confront him on his groping behavior. As if.

And my mother, my strikingly artistically gifted and intelligent mother who preferred to live in a surrealistic, made-up world of her own, trying to be my friend instead of my mother. She chose to believe my father and not me. As if. She told me that my panic attacks, which developed in the immediate aftermath of my father's first groping episode, were really sent by God as a dark night of the soul and meant I just needed to pray harder. As if.

As if anger is a bad thing. As if anger isn't protective, propelling, and proper in unjust situations.

As if I was right all along: I had been adopted. I firmly believed this as a child. I was born long after my siblings. My two childhood best friends were both adopted, and their parents didn't tell them this fact until they were older. I held a deep conviction that I was not of this family.

As if I was right all along: in order to survive, to heal, to thrive, I needed to sever ties, become unhomed, move far away to the Western frontier of Wallace Stegner's "native home of hope" and make my own way, my own family, my own home. What does it mean to be homeless when home was never a safe place? In such cases, it is not possible for young people to run away from home; they can only run towards home.

As if family secrets were legitimate heirlooms to pass down to future generations, squirreled away in cedar chests along with crocheted bedspreads and starched baby clothes.

My father never acknowledged his wrongdoing, never confessed his sins of groping me, of groping my maternal aunt when she was young, of groping at least one of his granddaughters. How can I begin to forgive him?

As if.

I spent many years of my adult life swinging wildly between minimizing the trauma ("It could have been worse") to full-body catastrophizing, drowning in the role of victim ("I am scarred and damaged beyond repair") before realizing that this is how our psyches cope with such trauma, and that the window of opportunity—for strength and hope and healing—lies in the space between those two extremes. It requires embracing the white-hot contradiction of the two truths. As if that were possible.

Until it is possible. Through a combination of fatigue, fortitude, and sheer inexplicable grace, it becomes possible.

But forgive? How can anyone forgive something as fundamentally wrong and psychically damaging as childhood sexual abuse by a parent? How can one forgive something that the perpetrator doesn't acknowledge having done, much less asked for forgiveness?

Learning that my father was sexually abused as a boy by his YMCA acrobatics coach does not lead me to forgive. As an adult he could have dealt with his own trauma so he wouldn't pass it on, like a genetic disorder, to his children and grandchildren. He didn't seek help, despite having the resources to do so; for that I do not forgive him. I do not forgive my mother for not believing me when I told her of the abuse. I do not forgive my siblings for the way they treated me after my father's death. I love them all, in that complicated, fierce, bloody rat's nest way of familial love. And I feel compassion for them, for the fear and the hurt and the grief they must have felt, and in the case of my siblings, still feel. But I don't forgive them.

I have come to forgive myself for not forgiving.

I recognize that not forgiving can lead to perpetual wallowing in victimhood, to anger, bitterness, unhappiness, physical and mental health problems. But it doesn't have to. It can be an act of charity and of self-respect.

Through forgiving oneself for not forgiving, much of the anger is channeled into sadness, into grief for what was missing in one's life, for evil in the world. Energy from the anger is transformed into the resolve to work to make things better for other people, as well as for oneself.

I recognize that our society does not forgive someone who does not forgive. Especially not a woman who does not forgive: she must be a freak of nature, a raging man-hating feminist. But, what would happen if I were to comply with societal expectations, force myself to preemptively and unilaterally forgive my father, absolve him of his wrongdoing? If he were still alive, it would convey to him that he had a free pass to continue his behavior unabated (which he did). And were he dead or alive, it would perpetuate male violence against women and children, and make our world less safe, less just (which it did). I have had times throughout my adult life when I sought to forgive my father and to try for some form of reconciliation. It never worked. It just opened me up to further abuse. And it allowed him to continue the cycle of abuse with younger female family members.

My father was aware of his transgressions. In one of his last years of life, when he was dying of congestive heart failure, he jokingly told me the story of a dream he'd had: he died and eagerly anticipated seeing my mother again, who had predeceased him. In his dream, he was greeted at the pearly gates by Saint Peter, who told him he couldn't go to heaven. Nor could he go to hell. So inside his dream he panicked and then awoke gasping for breath. When he told me of this dream—over the phone, with three thousand solid, safe miles between us—I knew that he was hovering close to acknowledging what he had done, yet he couldn't get to the point of confession, much less of asking for forgiveness. As I held the phone and listened, the familiar surreal cloud of dissociation gathered around me. But this time I didn't need the cloud to split my thinking-feeling self from my physical body. I felt anger but also profound sadness for my father, for his suffering.

"Dad, have you considered talking to your pastor about this?" I asked.

"Oh no, it's just a silly dream," he replied.

As far as I know, he never talked seriously with anyone, religious or otherwise, about his fears. But after that, when I visited him again in his home several weeks before he died, he once again said inappropriate sexual things to me and tried to fondle my breasts—this creepy, old, decrepit shell of a man. This time I was able not only to stop him, but also to say a final good-bye.

That was a year ago as I write this. Since it seems he was incapable of changing his ways, I am relieved my father is physically gone from my life, gone from this world. I have come to see that it is through speaking one's truth, and not through cheap, quick forgiveness, that we gain health and integrity. So often in our society we admonish people to mellow with age, to become more forgiving. I am now old enough to know better.

The scar is still there. The scar is an embodiment of what Donnel Stern terms "forgetful memory," or "anamnesis." It is there, yet it is beyond the mode of linear narrative. My experience of childhood trauma was something I could access solely through mosaic bits and pieces of poetry.

It is difficult but not impossible to find one's way to positive, non-self-destructive remembrance. I have found a way that doesn't overwhelm and send me spinning into a cloud of panic and dissociation. Remembrance that doesn't keep me in the perpetual ache of anger and righteous indignation. It involves learning to trust the body to remember, to trust that the scar will not rip open, all the while forging ahead. The way involves something more akin to resistance than resilience. There is a path to peace alongside truth, a path that does not require forgiveness, does not require forgetting. It is a path marked by the bruising bones of life.

Eleven

The Body Remembers

Let us turn our pain to power, our victimhood to fire, our self-hatred to action, our self-obsession to service, to fire, to wind.
—Eve Ensler

The Puget Sound tide here on Orcas Island is ebbing. I'm staying in a small cabin on a bluff overlooking Deer Harbor and Olga beach. Soon I'll take a break from my writing and walk the beach at low tide with my dog. I like to search for shards of smooth beach glass and pieces of old pottery from previous residents—long dead—of this tiny former fishing village. The tide goes out, revealing old artifacts. Tide out. Time out. Pausing and reflecting.

Where does it all go, the stress, the anger, the sting of old traumas? Where have all the panic attacks gone? The clouds of dissociation? The overwhelming sadness, the quicksand of ennui? How is it that words have carried me through? So many words. Words and stories give us a shareable world, but then, so do gestures, drawings, and photographs. What is so special about words?

The poet Adrienne Rich writes, "What kind of beast would turn its life into words? What atonement is this all about?—and yet, writing words like these I'm also living." In her poem "Cartographies of Silence" she also writes, "It was an old theme even for me: Language cannot do everything."

For over three decades of my life, I studied trauma. I studied the effects of trauma on young people and on communities. But I always studied trauma obliquely, safely, from within the cold confines of academia, with its distancing third-person voice. It was as if I could not admit to other people or to myself that I knew about this topic intimately and not just abstractly. This façade began to crumble through a combination of travel, teaching, reflective writing—and time.

I lived and worked in northern Thailand for much of the time between 2003 and 2006. For one of those years I had a Fulbright research and teaching award. I did research on Thai national policies and programs for homeless, street-involved children. I conducted in-person interviews with various people around the country, did site visits to programs aiding homeless children, and read the English-language Thai newspapers, listening for nuances of how language was used around these issues. I applied the research technique of discourse analysis, uncovering the connection between knowledge and power, and listening for evidence of Foucault's "counter-memories"—individual and collective memories that run counter to the "official" memories and histories of governments, mass media, and a society's power elite. Listening for the gaps, the silences, the pregnant pauses, the whispers "from within the shadows."

I learned that the main Thai term for street children in everyday conversation is *dek re ron*, with the literal translation being "child with no home" and closely aligned with the English-language terms *wanderer* and *vagrant*. One of the prevailing statements by the country's power elite was that the homeless street children were "not Thai people"—they were from the various Hill Tribe ethnic minority groups or were from the neighboring war-torn countries of Burma and Laos—and therefore they were not under the Bodhi tree protection of the king, the ultimate moral authority of Thailand.

I extended my research into an ethnography of the risk and protective factors affecting the health and well-being of a group of children living under bridges in Bangkok. Many of the children were forced into the country's extensive prostitution industry—an industry fueled by the presence of US troops in Thailand during the Vietnam War. And I taught community and psychiatric–mental health nursing to groups of nursing students from Seattle who lived and studied in Thailand for three months.

There is this from my notebook:

October 2006. I am sitting in a courtyard of an old wooden house in Chiang Mai, Thailand. There are blooming orchids all around me and the sweet smell of jasmine and the sound of falling water from a garden water feature—water spouting from a terracotta elephant's trunk off to my right side. I have been served oolong tea in a green Thai celadon tea set, another elephant's head and trunk forming the handle of my teacup. The teacup struck me as cloyingly sweet and touristy when I first saw it a few weeks ago, but it is growing on me and now strikes me as being supremely Thai in character. Perhaps I will buy one and take it home with me to Seattle. Then I can return to this courtyard whenever I sip tea from an elephant teacup. I can feel the same humid heat, the sweat trickling down my spine, smell the mixture of sweet jasmine and putrid *khlong* sewage, hear the tropical birds along with traffic sounds from the street—when I am sitting in my Seattle living room in winter gazing out at the rainy garden.

I am forced to revisit terrains of the soul that are painful, terrains littered with half-buried memories. Forced not just by travel and by living in a decidedly foreign country, but also forced by teaching mental health nursing here this quarter and having to discuss topics such as PTSD, eating disorders, and dissociation. I know I need to revisit these issues on a personal basis and be able to put them in some sort of perspective for myself, to know where they fit in to the person I am now—not so much to the person I was back when, back then. Although the past is present and who I was then is part of who I am now, and who I will become. I want to be able to be "real" and authentic and all those good things with my students, but not so much that I fall apart and cause them discomfort. That is a difficult line to walk, to be able to discern the difference between what is helpful to them and what is not.

I want to revisit the talk on surviving sexual abuse that I heard in New Orleans this past June at the National Health Care for the Homeless Conference. Things really clicked for me during her talk, things fell into place that hadn't before. I was able to see myself and know what had happened to me and how I had coped with it all these years. I was able to look at my past without falling apart or dissociating. How much of this do I ever really want to show the world? How much of this do I want to share with my students?

The conference workshop I refer to in this reflection was on trauma-informed care: health care provided within the framework of an understanding of the various neurocognitive, psychological, physiological, and social effects of trauma on individuals. People who are homeless have particularly high rates of trauma—both before and during their experience of homelessness. And, of course, homelessness itself is a type of trauma, a type of deep illness, as Arthur Frank calls is—an illness that casts a shadow over your life.

Trauma is an event that is life-threatening or "self" threatening. Serious accidents and medical mishaps. Drug and alcohol addictions. Natural and man-made disasters. Wars. Rapes. Intimate partner violence. Childhood neglect and physical and sexual abuse.

Complex trauma is trauma that occurs within key caretaker relationships and that is pervasive and enduring. Complex trauma is, well, more complex to live with and to treat.

We use the phrase "scared speechless" to describe fear that overwhelms and suppresses the speech and language area of our brains while we're in the midst of a traumatic event. As Bessel van der Kolk, a physician and expert on trauma, puts it, "All trauma is preverbal." Trauma bypasses these higher-order areas of the brain and goes straight to the more primitive fight-or-flight fear area—the amygdala, made of two almond-shaped areas deep inside our brains in the primitive limbic system.

Trauma is not stored as a storied memory with a clear-cut beginning, middle, and end, but rather as fragments of experience, images, smells, sounds, and other bodily sensations. That is why people who have survived a significant traumatic event struggle—even years and decades after the trauma is over—to be able to tell the story of what happened. Yet their bodies bear witness to the event through terrors, flashbacks, numbing, and stress-mediated physical problems like migraines and autoimmune diseases—diseases in which the body turns on itself, as if in slow suicide. If the trauma happened to the person as a child, before the firm development of a sense of self, that person's memories of the event can remain visceral and largely inaccessible to verbal processing.

Van der Kolk states that "almost every brain-imaging study of trauma patients finds abnormal activation of the insula. This part of the brain integrates and interprets the input from the internal organs—including our muscles, joints, and balance (proprioceptive) system—to generate the sense of being embodied." He points out that the flood of activating neurochemicals from the fight-or-flight response to trauma effectively cuts people off from the real origin of their bodily sensations: the fight-or-flight flood numbs people and is the reason for the dissociation and out-of-body experiences many trauma patients deal with. "In other words trauma makes people feel like *some body else*, or like *no body*. In order to overcome trauma, you need help to get back in touch with *your body*, with *your Self*."

Art, music, and dance are often used as treatments for trauma patients because these expressive modalities do not depend on language. They do not depend on—indeed, they are better off without—the use of our rational minds either to create or to experience. As psychiatrist Laurence J. Kirmayer writes, "And if the text stands for a hard-won rational order, imposed on thought through the careful composition of writing, the body provides a structure to thought that is, in part, extra-rational and disorderly. This extra-rational dimension to thought carries important information about emotional, aesthetic, and moral value."

In the late 1990s, in a Seattle-area community health clinic where I worked as a nurse practitioner, many of my patients were Bosnian and Ukrainian refugees. One of my more heart-wrenching experiences was with a four-year-old Bosnian girl whose teeth were rotted to the gum line because her mother had given her a sugar-soaked rag to suck in order to keep her silent as they tried to survive and then escape the civil war. The language interpreter told me that the child's older brother—and only sibling—had been killed, and that her mother had been raped.

I referred the child to our children's hospital, where they surgically removed all her baby teeth and then fitted her with child dentures to last until her adult teeth appeared. I was hoping to refer the mother for cultur-ally appropriate psychotherapy—"talk therapy"—to deal with her traumas, but soon realized it was best to refer her for massage therapy with a trauma-informed female therapist. I worked with our clinic social worker to petition the woman's health insurance (which happened to be the state Medicaid office) to pay for this—something typically considered slightly frivolous and self-indulgent treatment. Medicaid paid for the massage therapy, and it seemed to lighten her depression. This wasn't art, music, or dance therapy, but it was body-based therapy.

The body remembers. Maddy Coy, a UK-based researcher who works with survivors of prostitution, maintains that especially for women who experienced childhood sexual abuse (a startlingly high percentage of prostitutes worldwide), the use of appropriate body work such as yoga and massage is oftentimes crucial for recovery. Body work helps traumatized people reestablish a focus on what the body can do instead of what is and has been done to the body.

Early in my career as a nurse, I worked for a year in a "safe house" emergency shelter for women who were escaping intimate partner violence. Before my work there, I did not understand the concept of trauma mastery and how this plays out in the lives of women caught up in the cycle of abuse. I sided with the common misperception that the reason so many women return to their abusive partners is because the women are psychologically damaged and weak.

I learned that there is a not-insignificant role of addiction to the thrill of trauma and danger—to the effects of the very activating yet numbing fight-or-flight neurochemicals—which can bring at least temporary relief to the bouts of fatiguing depression that often accompany trauma. And there are also unconscious attempts to return to the site of previous trauma to "get it right this time"—to do what we wish we could have done the first time, to master our trauma.

Social worker Laura van Dernoot Lipsky points out that these unconscious attempts to master our traumas often backfire and simply reinforce our old traumas. She says that many of us in health care and other helping professions are often using our work as a type of trauma mastery, and that by doing so, we may set expectations for ourselves and others that are "untenable and destructive." She advocates ongoing efforts aimed at self-discovery and self-empathy, and points to the many positive examples of "people who have been effective in repairing the world while still in the process of repairing their own hearts." Eve Ensler, with the combination of personal work and "world repair" work that she describes in her powerful book *In the Body of the World*, is one of my favorite role models for this sort of balanced approach.

Language does appear to be important to the development of a healthy sense of self. We tend to believe that the ability to tell the story of, to narrate, our lives—whether or not we have experienced significant trauma—is a healthy and moral thing to do. There is a considerable body of research to support this claim. But there are also people, such as the philosopher Galen Strawson, who contest this notion. In his influential article "Against

Narrativity," Strawson distinguishes between people who are diachronic, who experience themselves with a past, present, and future—as having a storyline—and people who are (as Strawson claims himself to be) episodic, who experience themselves primarily in the here and now and not as having a grand storyline.

Strawson goes on to discuss the inherently faulty and messy nature of memory, claiming that people who tell stories of their lives are telling just that: stories, which are by necessity fabrications based loosely on facts. He concludes his essay with this discomfiting assertion: "As for Narrativity, it is in the sphere of ethics more of an affliction or a bad habit than a prerequisite of a good life. It risks a strange commodification of life and time—of soul, understood in a strictly secular sense."

The medical humanities scholar Angela Woods also warns that the privileging of narrative as inherently healthy, especially within the subfield of narrative medicine, functions to reproduce "Western, middle-class, liberal and neoliberal modes of being."

Contrary to the common cheery notion that telling our illness or trauma stories is salubrious, research shows that helping people piece together a story of what happened does not necessarily heal them, and that oftentimes their PTSD symptoms persist. Being able to tell the story of trauma—at least at some level and in whatever form—may be necessary for healing, but it isn't sufficient. Having a coherent story of trauma can help us through certain rough patches in life, but it can also become detrimental, especially when it cannot be adapted to changing circumstances, or when it becomes a broken record of woe-is-me victimhood. As Arthur Frank reminds us, telling one's own illness or trauma narrative is important, but it can become singular and claustrophobic unless it opens one up to more universal connections with other people and with the world.

And then there is the danger that Louise DeSalvo writes about in her book *Writing as a Way of Healing: How Telling Our Stories Transforms Our Lives*:

> The dilemma writers face is that though writing an organized, well-structured piece of work helps us integrate trauma into our lives, writing an organized, well-structured piece of work about extreme experiences seems (is) unethical and immoral. If we present such experiences as if they

can be subsumed into coherent, orderly aesthetic objects, aren't we ourselves participating in the misapprehension of these experiences? in their misrepresentation?

Telling the story of trauma—of survival—may have the capacity to at least aid in healing at the individual level, but then there is the added danger, once the story is shared, of it being appropriated and misused by more powerful political or fundraising causes. Stories can be stolen. Arthur Frank calls these "hijacked narratives"—"Telling one's own story is good, but it is never inherently good, and the story is never entirely one's own."

An intriguing example of a stolen story is the one explored in Rebecca Skloot's narrative nonfiction book *The Immortal Life of Henrietta Lacks*, a book that tells the story of the cervical cancer cells "stolen" from an impoverished and poorly educated black woman in Baltimore in the 1950s. Scientists at Johns Hopkins Hospital subsequently profited from culturing and selling these HeLa cells—cells which killed Henrietta Lacks, cells which neither she nor her family members consented to anyone using or profiting from. Skloot, a highly educated white woman, has also now profited from the use of the Lacks' family story, although she has set up a scholarship fund for the Lacks family members.

I am reminded of the proverb that Vanessa Northington Gamble shares in her moving essay, "Subcutaneous Scars," written about her experience of racism as a black physician. Dr. Gamble's grandmother, a poor black woman in Philadelphia, used to admonish her, "The three most important things that you own in this world are your name, your word, and your story. Be careful who you tell your story to."

The body remembers; my body remembers, I think to myself, as I sit in a hot tub beside my cabin on Orcas Island. *Where did all these scars come from? What stories do my scars tell?* I wonder, as I inventory my scars. From the slight dent in my left forehead from crawling out of my crib and falling on the corner of a bookcase sometime in my infancy, to the more recent white, jagged scar on my right pinky toe from dropping a heavy garden pot on it a year ago. There they are, my assortment of scars. I study a long, faint, white scar on my left shin, remember gouging myself there as a young teenager while trying to learn to shave my legs.

But as I stare at this pale spot, I begin to remember fragments of an earlier injury there, from the summer I turned four. My friend Suzie, who was my same age, and I were playing in the woods near my house when our fathers came running towards us, yelling in anger about the fact that we had left our families, who were camping nearby. Suzie and I ran into my house in search of shelter. I quickly climbed into an upper, hidden part of the closet of my bedroom, scraping my left shin on an exposed nail. I stifled my urge to scream. As I hid there in the closet, bleeding, I heard Suzie's screams and cries from my parents' bedroom where our fathers were jointly spanking her, but which she told me—years later when we were young adults and which I at some level already knew—went much further than just spanking.

Yes, this continuous flow of stories of trauma and of childhood abuse is difficult to listen to. Yes, dear reader, I know that. But as long as they continue to happen, especially at such high rates, I believe we need to increase our capacity to listen, to hear, and to work to change the conditions that allow such things to continue.

Staring now at this scar on my shin, I remember searing pain, combined with absolute fear, tinged with an overlay of stultifying guilt from my inability to try to intervene, somehow, to help my friend. As if I could have done that at age four. And now, my eureka moment in this oh-so-West-Coast hot tub is that several months following this incident, I began having vivid and recurring rescue dreams consisting of me being on a tricycle at kindergarten (which Suzie also attended, in real life as well as in my dream) and suddenly pedaling furiously to the aid of an injured classmate who'd gotten hit by a car. Has my career been at least partially driven by wanting to return to that closet, this time to climb out, somehow transformed into a fierce, adult, and kind-hearted Nurse Ratched who sends our abusive fathers flying?

But this complex, mostly preverbal and visceral, memory of trauma remains stubbornly in a liminal, threshold place—a place of uncertainty and dis-ease. Learning how to leave it there, to live with it, to trust that the body remembers this largely mute and silent history of mine, to recognize that it will always be a part of me but never essentially me—that is the wisdom worth searching for. Indeed, it occurs to me that it is what I am searching for when I collect all the broken shards of pottery and sea-smoothed glass on the beach at low tide.

Twelve

Endurance Test

... this fevered exploration of both the psychological cost of paying attention to the tragedies of others and the social cost of looking away.
—Katherine Boo

What helps us—as health care providers, as caregivers, as people, as communities—to endure the various traumas and sufferings that we're exposed to indirectly and that we experience ourselves?

Resilience is something that is often cited as an answer to this question. *Resilience* is a term adapted from engineering to describe the ability of a substance, such as a metal, to return to its previous state after being stressed—the substance is able to bounce back, to return to steady state, to normal. The American Psychological Association's definition of *resilience* is "the process of adapting well in the face of adversity, trauma, tragedy, threats or even significant sources of threat." Resilience is sometimes referred to as "good survival."

Over the past several decades, there has been an explosion of research on resilience, mainly focusing on individual risk and protective factors. The main protective factors are, not surprisingly, (1) the formation of a firm, secure attachment to a parent or caretaker figure within the first few years of life; (2) prosocial behaviors and personality traits, such as empathy, a positive attitude, capacity for forgiveness, and ability to "play well with others"; and (3) a sense of personal agency, of being able to act, to do something positive both in the midst and the wake of trauma. The main risk factors are, not surprisingly, the opposite of the protective factors.

Most research on resilience has focused on the individual, is Western-centric, and has increasingly become biologically reductionist, narrowing in on the epigenetics of trauma and resilience, finding individuals and entire communities of people with "short alleles" and DNA methylation—genetic markers of increased vulnerability to the adverse effects of trauma. That these are most often individuals and communities already marginalized by poverty and racism and other socially constructed vulnerabilities serves to further label and pathologize people and communities. It marks them as damaged goods. As irredeemably, permanently damaged goods. It typically ignores the mounting research evidence indicating that such epigenetic damage is largely reversible and preventable with appropriate life experiences—with access to appropriate life experiences, including effective therapeutic interventions.

Resilience-building interventions include cognitive-behavioral psychotherapy; therapies focused on building the capacity for empathy and forgiveness; narrative storytelling and other meaning-making therapies; and therapies aimed at increasing social support—social support that includes social touch, the human version of primate grooming. Good touch: a handshake, a peck on the cheek, or a hug in greeting; a hand brushing a shoulder in sympathy; sitting close to a stranger on a bus; washing the feet of people who are homeless, people who are rarely touched in a good way.

This all sounds good, but resilience irritates me. The whole saccharine notion that the human body, the human psyche, and even entire communities can be like heated metal—stressed and stretched but not broken—that they can bounce back, return to steady state, and perhaps be stronger and wiser for the experience? Certainly I believe that strength-based research and interventions are an important and sizeable improvement over the traditional deficit models so prevalent within health and social services. But resilience has its dark side.

Resilience tends to glorify trauma. It contributes to an addiction to pain and to suffering. *What doesn't kill you makes you stronger. Be the hero of your own life. Cancer saved my life, made me a better person.* "The world breaks everyone," said Hemingway, "and afterward, some are strong at the broken places." Resilience glosses over the fact that trauma and resilience are not equal opportunity affairs, that some people (women, children, people with various disabilities, nonwhite people, and gender-nonconforming people) and some communities (those marginalized by homelessness, poverty, racism, and the effects of colonization) are much more likely to be exposed to traumas in the first place, and they have fewer resources for weathering and recovering from trauma. Resilience ignores the larger structural inequities, as well as the stigmatizing narratives we place on certain people, communities, and entire impoverished countries. As physician, anthropologist, and global health champion Paul Farmer reminds us, "The capacity to suffer is, clearly, part of being human. But not all suffering is equal, in spite of pernicious and often self-serving identity politics that suggest otherwise."

Trauma never happens in isolation. Even if it is a one-time trauma that occurs to one individual, trauma happens within the context of a particular family, community, and cultural, social, and time period. An individual trauma ripples outward as well as inward. Suffering from trauma is always a social process; recovering from trauma is always a social process. If suffering is a universal yet unequal human experience, the ability to tell and listen to illness and trauma narratives matters. But it doesn't stop there. Physician, anthropologist, and expert on illness narratives Arthur Kleinman admonishes us that it is the moral and emotional cores of these experiences that matter much more, including the cores of social suffering that especially affect marginalized people.

Kleinman also encourages us to ask the question, "What helps us endure?"

> And I mean by endure withstand, live through, put up with, and suffer. I do not mean the currently fashionable and superficially optimistic idea of "resilience" as denoting a return to robust health and happiness. Those who have struggled in the darkness of their own pain or loss, or that of patients or loved ones, know that these experiences, even when left behind, leave traces that may only be remembered viscerally but shape their lives beyond.

Trauma and resilience occur at the community level. Manhattan after the 9/11 World Trade Center attacks. The 2004 tsunami in the Indian Ocean. The 2011 Tohoku earthquake, tsunami, and nuclear disaster in Japan. The series of earthquakes in Christchurch, New Zealand, also in 2011. In the United States, the still-reverberating effects of trauma and social suffering from slavery and from the treatment of Native Americans. And, of course, more recent national disgraces such as what happened in New Orleans in 2005 with Hurricane Katrina: the perfect storm of a simultaneous natural and man-made disaster that highlighted entrenched racism, classism, and environmental degradation.

New Orleans, a city of trauma and survival, has long held a fascination for me. I first visited New Orleans in June 1977, a few days after I turned seventeen. I stayed in the city for several days with a church youth group that I was part of. We were on our way to do a summer-long missionary trip in rural Mexico. Spinning off from the main group, I had my first mixed drink (a cloyingly sweet Hawaiian Sunrise—which must have sounded exotic and sophisticated to me then) in a bar on Bourbon Street. Walking along the streets, I giggled as I furtively glanced at garish female prostitutes hanging their body parts from balconies. I was evicted by police from a town fountain that I was splashing in while trying to cool off from the oppressively muggy summer weather.

From rereading my travel journal, I see that this was a trip in which I dealt with relationships with various boys in my life, frequent gastrointestinal illnesses, a nasty scorpion bite, and nighttime panic attacks which I discreetly referred to in my journal as "the fear" without describing it in any detail—for fear of the fear. I didn't yet know they were properly called panic attacks, and I certainly didn't know where they came from at that point in my life.

The next time I was in New Orleans was in late June 2004, for the National Health Care for the Homeless Conference, during which I wrote the following reflection:

The plane landed between potholes and mud puddles on the thin strip of concrete—skidding languorously to a stop, splattering more rain on the cabin windows. The mud would be a constant theme throughout my week-long stay in New Orleans, this island swamp city. Inside the airport and then on the downtown streets, the people have an island, Caribbean look: ebony and café au lait skin, beads of sweat above every lip. The sweat here is not just on the surface of the skin; it seeps down inside, down the trachea, making me cough constantly. Afternoon thunderstorms sneak up and slide down the muddy Mississippi, suddenly clanging overhead in a single clap like the starting note of a brass band, followed by torrents of warm rain.

It can't be easy being homeless in this town of swamp mud, sweat, rain, and river water. I have a hard time telling who is homeless and who is not. The tourists are easy to spot, with their big bellies girded by fanny packs, as if they are strolling around Disneyland. But everyone else defies my classification. Outside the French Quarter A&P, which contains at least ten varieties of grits, I search for the homeless youth I have been told congregate near the store. If they are here I don't see them and they certainly don't look like the West Coast homeless young people I am used to seeing and working with. Outside the store is a large black man in starched new denim overalls, a pork-pie hat, and sporting a voluminous white beard. He sits on a gray plastic milk crate and plays a harmonica hidden somewhere inside the beard. Between sets he talks to people going by who he seems to know, and sometimes he stops playing, stands on top of the crate, and gazes over the crowd, as if looking for someone.

The nighttime cockroaches that scurry up out of sidewalk cracks startle me at first, and then they become strangely reassuring—reassuring because this Southern swamp city has to have cockroaches.

Cockroaches and tourists I can spot on New Orleans's streets, but the homeless young people continue to elude me. I've spent my whole adult life working with "street kids" from all over the country. On this trip I've spent some time in downtown New Orleans at a youth drop-in center with its local black kids mixing uneasily with the mostly white, scruffy-looking young people who call themselves "urban nomads." Mainly young men. They're just passing through town with backpacks and piercings and tattoos, pretending to be modern-day versions of Jack Kerouac. New Orleans is the big party-town stop on their circuit.

I begin to discern these same—or similar—young people along the streets and in the parks. None of them are "spanging," asking for spare change. They all either play various musical instruments, or they sit at impromptu booths doing tarot card or palm readings. No one has asked me for change. No one—young or old—is begging on the streets of New Orleans. Perhaps it is illegal in this town? Perhaps the notoriously harsh city police keep it from happening? Or perhaps there's enough music and magic in the city to feed everyone?

With that last phrase, I realized that I was caught up in the heavily romanticized and sanitized storyline of New Orleans that the city's tourist bureau likes to peddle—of the resilient "poor black folks" from New Orleans who persevere and overcome through the use of their rich musical heritage.

I returned to New Orleans in May 2014 to attend the National Health Care for the Homeless Conference & Policy Symposium once again—it is one of my favorite conferences. The last time I'd been in New Orleans was in 2005, less than two months before Hurricane Katrina tried to return it to the sea. In Seattle, in the first few years after Katrina, I had taken care of many homeless and near-homeless patients who had been displaced by the storm. I knew that most of these community clinic patients were among the more than one hundred thousand former residents of New Orleans who left in the aftermath of Katrina—never to return.

Now, almost a decade after the devastating hurricane and the national tragedy of how it was handled, I wondered how the citizens of New Orleans had chosen to remember it. I went back to New Orleans to participate in the conference, but also to track down residents' Katrina memorials, their collective sites of memory. How individuals and communities deal with the aftermath of a large-scale disaster was something I'd been pondering, especially since I had recently returned from New Zealand, where I sought to understand some of the effects of the earthquakes on Christchurch residents. How do people deal with and bear witness to trauma? How do people, how do entire communities, deal with and bear witness to the complex and nuanced layers of trauma?

When I arrived in New Orleans, I knew that there was a Katrina National Memorial Park, but I wasn't exactly sure where it was located. When I asked the concierge at the conference hotel, he said he had never heard of it, and he had to do an internet search to find it. I took a lumbering streetcar northwest on Canal Street towards the Cities of the Dead, the city's famous series of aboveground cemeteries—above ground since the city is below sea level and the buried bodies would otherwise float to the surface. The new Katrina memorial was located in one of these old Cities of the Dead.

It was late afternoon when I arrived at the black iron gates marked "Katrina National Memorial." Giant white-and-gray thunderheads were billowing higher and higher in the sky, accompanied by the distant rattle of thunder. Entering the black wrought-iron gates, I read the first sign, telling me this was the site of the Charity Hospital Cemetery, on land purchased by

Charity Hospital in 1848, and called Potter's Field in the lingo of the time. "It has historically been used to bury the unclaimed from throughout the city, including the victims of several yellow fever and influenza epidemics," proclaims the sign.

Walking farther into the cemetery—alone, I saw no other people while I was there—I was greeted by a series of large, shiny, rectangular black marble structures, which another sign identified as the Katrina Memorial mausoleums. They contain the ashes of the dead—all those dead bodies that were found yet not identified, or if identified, never claimed by relatives. These mausoleums bear a strong resemblance to the nondescript yet menacing boxcars the Germans used to transport Jews, the homeless, gays, Gypsies, and other "undesirables" to concentration camps and gas chambers. A sign states that the swirling pathways lined with these strange structures are supposed to mimic the shape of the hurricane. It is designed to "create a meditative labyrinth, a healing space for reflection." This space, this site of memory, was neither meditative nor healing. Who, I wondered, was responsible for the design of this place?

Ah, of course! I thought, as I read a sign stating that this Katrina memorial was created by "Dr. Frank Minyard, Coroner of Orleans Parish." I already knew that Dr. Minyard was an obstetrics/gynecology physician by training, a white man dubbed "Dr. Jazz" as well as "friend of the police"—for his love of both trumpet playing and covering up controversial "accidental" deaths of black men and poor people while in police custody. As I sat on a bench waiting for the Streetcar Not Named Desire back to my French Quarter tourist hotel, I felt sad, empty, and duped.

Having visited and been disappointed by the Katrina National Memorial Park, I decided to visit the permanent exhibit *Living with Hurricanes: Katrina and Beyond*, located at the Presbytère Louisiana State Museum in the heart of the French Quarter. Greeting me in a wildly disorienting way as I entered the main door of the museum building was an art installation: *Message of Remembrances* (2010), by Mitchell Gaudet. Hundreds of "floating" glass bottles with messages curled up inside them, all hanging from the ceiling. Interspersed among the bottles were ghostly blue glass hands, reaching down—or wait! were they reaching up, out of the deluge, the person attached to the hand drowning and asking to be rescued? I stood in the middle of the foyer gazing up at the display as the lights surrounding it gyrated from blue to purple to pink to red and back again, trying to figure out which way was up and which was down. Who are the rescuers and who are the rescued? It felt as if I were simultaneously the rescuer and the rescued—floating in the psychedelic, primordial sea of life.

The bottle installation also reminded me of that uniquely Southern folk art of bottle trees, as captured in an iconic image by the venerable Southern writer and Works Progress Administration photographer Eudora Welty. A black-and-white photograph of a shack of a house in Mississippi with a large bottle tree on the bare-earth front yard. The folk belief is that placing bottles on trees away from the main entrance to the house will help to capture and repel bottle genies, djinn, or haints—spirits that haunt a place. The bottle trees are thought to protect people and their homes from calamities. Maybe all the pent-up bottle djinn in the New Orleans area had been released by Katrina, and the artist of this installation was trying to once again contain them.

At the entrance to the Katrina exhibit was a large sign: "Resilience." *Oh no, here we go again with the officially scripted, up-with-people resilience narrative*, I thought, as I entered the darkened room. I will attempt to suspend my critical stance and give this museum exhibit on Katrina an honest chance, I told myself.

As I snaked my way through the rooms of the exhibit, I found quite a lot to admire in how the curators had chosen to tell the story of and to commemorate Katrina. The first few rooms were dark and immersive, showing billowing smoke from one downtown New Orleans building next to a display of an ax stored in the attic of a mock house—the ax being an essential home safety precaution in that many people during Katrina were trapped inside their attics by the rising water and drowned because they couldn't chop an escape route through their roofs.

Then I entered the second room of the exhibit, filled with separate displays about "ordinary heroes": hospital nurses and physicians, first responders, and citizens who volunteered to help during and after the disaster. The displays included seats from the Superdome fiasco, samples of emergency cans of water from the Red Cross, and military MREs (meals ready to eat) that included little bottles of Tabasco hot sauce. There was one brief and somewhat sanitized display labeled "Race, Class, and Inequality," with a heavily edited quote from then president George W. Bush. This second room was filled with random flashing lights of red, yellow, and that freaky blue again, echoing the bottle display in the foyer.

There was quite a lot of content on the effects of climate change, environmental degradation, and engineering mistakes, which all compounded the devastation of Hurricane Katrina. In this section, audio-recordings of Katrina survivors played in an endless loop. An African American man, a former resident of the most severely affected Ninth Ward district, had this to say: "The water in the vast area matched the speed of a second hand of a clock—that was the amount of time it took for that water to rise. I don't remember hearing it before: a sound like a freight train." I found his first-person testimony both eloquent and haunting, and I listened to the loop several times to make sure I wrote down his exact words.

But one section of the Katrina exhibit has continued to disturb me. It takes up the most space in the middle part of the exhibit, being eight or nine panels, sections of the actual walls of a central New Orleans housing-project apartment. The walls preserve the wall diary of Tommie Elton Mabry, who was in his early fifties at the time of Katrina. He called it his "ledger or graffiti," which he wrote with a black Sharpie pen. Mabry, who had been homeless "since Regan was president," as he put it to a reporter, took refuge from the approaching storm in a first-floor apartment in the deserted high-rise B. W. Cooper public housing development in downtown New Orleans. He stayed in the apartment from the day before Hurricane Katrina hit New Orleans until two months later, when he was forced to leave by the housing authority officials. The building has since been torn down, but city officials decided to keep and preserve his original wall diary.

What bothers me about this part of the exhibit are the unacknowledged—the silenced—ethical issues, power dynamics, and inherent racism and classism within it. Mabry's diary entries are written in about a fourth- or fifth-grade level and include frequent f-bombs. Many of the entries focus on him getting drunk or nursing a hangover. These all highlight negative stereotypes of homeless people, and especially of African Americans living in poverty and homelessness. In the photos included in the museum display, and in several local newspaper articles, Mabry appears to be proud of the fact that his diary is now on permanent display in a New Orleans museum. But did anyone bother to ask his permission before they preserved his wall diaries? Did anyone consider setting up some sort of appropriate payment to him, for instance a housing or health fund, for the use of his words, his story? Did they not pay him because he wrote his Katrina diary on the walls of a public housing unit, which were not rightfully his to own or to profit from?

Tommie Elton Mabry died of a heart attack in 2013, at the age of fifty-eight. He was still homeless and couch-surfing in New Orleans at the time of his death.

Resilience, either for an individual or a community—even if it were possible, would it be desirable? If most traumas, most disasters, are at least partially caused by and certainly compounded by social (in)justice issues, do we want to "return to normal," to the status quo, after our worlds, our bodies, our communities have been shaken to the foundations, have been flooded by mud, have been seared by fire, have been permanently altered and scarred? Skirting close to the danger of glorifying trauma, of feeding an addiction to the pain and suffering so overly abundant in our world, is the recognition that individual and community healing "means repair but it also means transformation—transformation to a different moral state." And it means enduring, going on, doing what we can individually and collectively to transform the world for the better.

Thirteen

An Overexamined Life

Coming home at last
At the end of the year,
I wept to find
My old umbilical cord.
—Basho

Sunday, December 13, 2015. Orcas Island, Washington. 7:00 a.m. My last full day here. I've already started packing my things and will take them to the car trunk today if it ever stops raining.

As I begin writing this essay, at the end of a week-long solo writing retreat in a tiny cabin on an island near my home, I also begin writing in a new journal, a simple black-and-white composition notebook. It is the 122nd journal I have written so far in my life. Or perhaps it is my 123rd journal, as I lost one I wrote back in the fall of 1989 through 1990, the year I was working my way into and then out of homelessness, the year I lived in so many places I lost count.

It is a significant gap, both in my memory and in my journal writing. I wish I had that specific journal. Most likely, I left it behind in some random short-term boyfriend's place. There were a fair number of them back then— the boyfriends, not the journals—something of which I am neither proud nor ashamed. The fact that my life was so chaotic that I lost my journal, the recording of my life during that time, is in itself emblematic of what happens with too much rootlessness, too much home-less-ness.

I now live in my own house in Seattle, which this year has become the one home I have lived in for the longest period of my life: nineteen years. I lived in my rural Virginia childhood home from the time I was born until I left for college at age eighteen. I mention this because while my journal writing began in my Virginia home when I was twelve, it became an essential part of my life somewhere along the way. And it seems to have picked up in intensity during the years I've lived in my current home, my own home, with a mortgage I've almost finished paying off.

This past spring, I was deeply into a serious cleaning, into reducing my physical belongings, the detritus of life. One advantage of the rootlessness of frequent moves is that this "sort and purge" occurs more frequently. Plus, in the year since my father died, I was left with boxes of his detritus—and that of my mother, who predeceased him—that I now had to deal with.

Compounding the urgency of this particular spring cleaning was the fact that my then twenty-seven-year-old son had broken up with his girlfriend and precipitously moved back into his childhood bedroom. The bedroom closet of which contained all of my old journals. I wasn't ready for my son to stumble upon and read them. If I'll ever be ready for that. How much do we want our children, no matter what their age, to know about us? So, I was forced to think of legacy, of what's left behind when people die, of what I don't want my son to have to deal with after I am gone. Assuming it goes that way, the natural order of things. Being the one at the end of the diving board of life does change one's perspective on many aspects of life and of living.

I removed my journal collection from his closet and counted them: 119 journals at that point. Then I stacked them on the floor of my office and covered the pile with a blanket, as if for protection. Every morning when I sipped coffee and wrote in my current journal, I contemplated the now shrouded journal corpse in the corner of the room. This growing pile of journals: Should I keep them? Burn them?

Why did I—why does anyone—write and keep journals? What is this urge to narrate, to record, to leave written artifacts of a life? What do people decide to do with all their journals, and why? What are the limits to such an examined life, and when does it become an overexamined life?

Monday, December 14, 2015. Orcas Island, Washington. 6:30 a.m. The sun, such as it is, is slowly rising. I can now discern the dark outlines of the islands versus the lighter midnight blue of the water of Puget Sound. I love this time of year. So moody and introverted and brooding.

The *Oxford English Dictionary* states that the word *journal* derives from the Latin *diurnal*, meaning "of or belonging to a day," and from Old French *jur*—meaning "surroundings/vicinity"—and *el*, "daily." A day's work; a measure of land that can be plowed in a day; a record of travel; a record of business accounts; a breviary, or collection of daily prayers; a daily newspaper or "public journal," as in the *Wall Street Journal.* "A record of events of personal interest—entries are made day by day or as events occur." *Diary* is from the Latin *diarium*: daily allowance or journal. Journal and diary are typically used interchangeably at the current time, at least in the United States, although historically, "diary" seems to have been the preferred term.

From a University of Washington (UW, my current employer) library search, I find a dizzying array of types of journals. Reflective practice journals. Therapeutic journals. Journals to teach children and adults writing skills or a second language. Spiritual practice, Bible, and prayer journals. Gratitude journals. Dream journals. Travel journals. Behavioral change, such as weight loss, journals. Grief and bereavement journals. Illness journals. Trauma journals. Artist's and writer's journals. Professional development journals, like the ones used for medical, nursing, and counseling students. And, of course, all of those academic discipline journals through which I am now learning these facts.

Blogging can be a form of public journaling. And there are computer and mobile phone apps for journaling so there is no hassle with using pen and paper. Online journaling sites are either private, with declarations such as "military grade security," or shareable and public. One of these online journaling sites, Journalate, has the intriguing tagline "Empty your head. Privately." A journal as a dumping ground container (like a toilet) for raw emotions.

Cabins have journals—like the Orcas Island one I was staying in when I began writing this essay. On my last day there, I read through this cabin journal. Honeymooning couples, families with small children, a mother grieving the loss of her youngest child. The chirpy, exclamation-pointed, flowery-script entries. The painfully raw "TMI" stories. The lists of things to do or not do, see or not see, left by well-intentioned visitors. "Make sure to hike Mt Constitution or visit the beach at low tide and check out the starfish." Silly entries written from the perspective of a person's dog. Weather reports. Quite a few entries about it being rainy and windy, as it was during my stay. Admonishments to watch out for dive-bombing owls nesting in trees outside.

Closing the cabin journal without having written in it, I was aware of the lingering effects of whispering ghosts and glad I hadn't read it earlier in my stay. I wondered, what motivates people to write in these sorts of communal journals? Perhaps it is akin to carving one's initials on trees: I was here. I exist. I matter. To connect with the line of other people who have—and who will—inhabit this space, sleep in this bed, gaze at this view of Puget Sound.

Tuesday, December 15, 2015. Seattle, Washington. 8:30 a.m. Ah. Back home. I have library books at UW to pick up. There were four hundred email messages in my UW account when I got home. All but five I instantly deleted. I feel drawn back into the chatter of the world.

What are some of the earliest examples of journals? Augustine's Confessions perhaps, assuming he based his spiritual autobiography on some sort of journal or diary. I pause to read this work of his, written around AD 400, and find that in book 4, after describing his grief over the death of a male friend—and a digression into a consideration of what is beautiful—there's this fascinating statement: "I wrote 'on the fair and fit' I think two or three books. Thou knowest, O Lord, for it is gone from me; for I have them not, but they are strayed from me, I know not how." Did Augustine lose some of his journals, his books, and in this passage mourn their loss along with the loss of his friend, as if they were both parts of himself?

On the opposite side of the world, the Japanese poet Basho spent almost a decade of his life, between 1683 and 1691, on solo hiking trips around Japan, during which he wrote his travel journals in *haibun*, a combination of prose and haiku. He took the first of his travels after his home burned down, followed soon after by the death of his mother. In *Travels of a Travelworn Satchel*, which includes his now famous haiku and the epigraph of this essay, Basho reflects on the keeping of a travel diary, and he writes, "My records are little more than the babble of the intoxicated and the rambling talk of the dreaming."

There are the journals of explorers and scientists, overwhelmingly written by men (Marie Curie a notable exception). Benjamin Franklin, Thomas

Jefferson, Alexis de Tocqueville, Charles Darwin, Leonardo da Vinci, Sir Isaac Newton, Thomas Edison, the Chinese geographer Hsu Hsia-k'o, Christopher Columbus, Captain James Cook, Meriwether Lewis and William Clark. Then there is Captain Robert F. Scott's logbook journal of his final exploration of Antarctica, where he and his entire party died on their way back and weren't discovered—with the frozen but readable journals—until eight months later. One of his last journal entries: "These rough notes and our dead bodies must tell the tale …"

Both Thomas Jefferson and Benjamin Franklin carried pocket notebooks made of thin ivory leaves held together by brass or silver fittings, the leaves opening in a fan shape. They wrote on the leaves with a pencil, transferred the notes to paper ledgers at the end of the day, and then erased the pencil marks with a moist finger so the ivory notebook could be used again. Franklin even had such a notebook specially made with days of the week and his virtues written on each page.

I carry a five-by-eight-inch Moleskine notebook with me wherever I go and use it to write random thoughts, project ideas, small sketches, and bits of conversation from people around me. Some content finds its way into my journal entries the next day. I now have a shelf-full of these notebooks, all filled with my wonderings and wanderings—but not my virtues. They are the perfect size to stash in my purse or bike bag. But now I am fascinated by these antique ivory-leafed tiny pocket notebooks, and discover that a small company in Indiana sells replicas made of brass and repurposed ivory piano keys.

I consider purchasing one. It has a hasp to allow it to be worn on a chain around one's neck or attached to a belt. It would go nicely with a little silver pencil pendant I inherited from my maternal great-grandmother, who loved to write but was given the famous female-only "rest cure" of Gilman's *The Yellow Wallpaper*, and wasn't allowed to read or write for days at a time. I inherited her pencil pendant and a fragment of her diary containing this pithy comment: "I have been near insanity and devil possession induced by two antique hounds and their accursed visitations."

There are those (mostly women) who made a business of, or at least became famous for, journal writing. Anne Frank. Anaïs Nin and her seven volumes of published journals. May Sarton. Katherine Mansfield. Simone de Beauvoir. And closer to my Seattle home, Ivan Doig and his book *Winter*

Brothers: A Season at the Edge of America, in which he combined the diaries of the Pacific Northwest pioneer James G. Swan with his own journal entries.

Doig was a historian at home in the dusty UW archives where he discovered Swan's diaries, which Swan kept for forty years that—by Doig's calculations—resulted in 2.5 million words by hand. In Winter Brothers, Doig writes,

> Swan's day-upon-day sluice of diary words: why? Was the diarying habit something which surfaced out of instinct, the unslakable one that murmurs in some of us that our way to put a mark on the world is not with the sword or tool, but pen? Or did contents mean more to him than the doing of it—the diary a way to touch out into life as it flowed past him and skim the most interesting as an elixir? … Swan works at these pages of his as steadily, incessantly, as a man building a castle out of pebbles.

Historians such as Doig, as well as scholars in other fields, use personal journals as primary sources to build a case for whatever theory they have about the person, about events, or about the time period within which the person was writing. One of the most famous of these is the decade-long, million-word diary written by the seventeenth-century British civil servant Samuel Pepys. In his diaries, written in shorthand and coded for the juicier sections, he writes of his everyday life, of his extramarital affairs, and of politics. He records that when he was forced to evacuate his home during the Great Fire of London, he sent his journals, along with other items of personal value, ahead of him to safety. Historians have used his diaries to help piece together details of both the Great Fire and the Great Plague of London, as well as of what daily life was like for an upper-middle-class Londoner during the decade of the 1660s. Journals as scholarly clues.

Journals as clues to deaths. Police and forensics experts search quickly for personal diaries or journals to help piece together the story of what happened, to provide answers to questions: Who wanted to kill a person, and why? Did they want to kill themselves, and why?

Wednesday, December 16, 2015. Seattle, Washington. 8:00 a.m. I got so much writing and work done out on Orcas Island, it's a bit frustrating returning home to way too many distractions—email and chores and Christmas preparations.

Journals are typically written in the first-person singular "I," sometimes in the form of an imagined letter to someone, or to an imagined someone. My first journal entries at age twelve always started with "Dear Dragon," as I had an imaginary fire-breathing friend who was my fierce protector. More rarely, journals are written in the distancing stance of third person. Although, as Thoreau states in his introduction to *Walden*, "We commonly do not remember that it is, after all, always the first person that is speaking." Thoreau knew what he was talking about. Between 1837 and 1861, Thoreau wrote daily in his journal, accumulating seven thousand pages of cryptically handwritten entries, all in first person.

Diaries and journals are typically solo affairs, but there are examples of couples who write in a shared journal—why? Is this a healthy practice or a sign of emotional enmeshment, as it seems to have been for the shared diaries of Leo Tolstoy and his wife, Sonya? And is that latter notion an indication of my own harsh cynicism and judgmentalism because I cannot imagine ever writing in a couple's journal?

But wait. I remember now that I tried keeping a couple's journal more than a decade ago, along with my partner, upon the advice of a couple's counselor. We had intimacy issues in our relationship, having both endured rocky divorces and each having a child from our previous marriages. My partner wrote one entry on the first page of our journal, an entry I responded to promptly in writing. But that was it. He stopped writing. Not wanting to waste a perfectly good composition notebook, it became my own journal. The couple's journal died, but that coupled partnership survived. I think it has something to do with me having the space and trust within my relationship that allow for the keeping of a private journal.

Thursday, December 17, 2015. Seattle, Washington. 9:00 a.m. Raining. My days have been too disjointed since I returned—too many distractions. I need to do a big clean, upstairs and downstairs. Get rid of clutter and dust and cobwebs. I haven't been able to keep up the writing momentum I was into while out on Orcas. Frustrating. I hope I can get back into it soon, but with the holidays approaching, that may not be possible. Balance. I need family time as well as work/writing time.

Writing of any sort, including a personal journal, is a luxury, a privilege we often take for granted. It requires access to basic education, writing implements, and the time, space, and solitude in which to write. Journal writing is not an equal opportunity endeavor. In Tillie Olsen's now classic feminist short story "I Stand Here Ironing," the protagonist, a working-class mother, as was Olsen, thinks to herself, "And when is there time to remember, to sift, to weigh, to estimate, to total? I will start and there will be an interruption and I will have to gather it all together again."

Those of us who are mothers—still—in modern-day, marginally more egalitarian, and less-prone-to-ironing twenty-first-century America, can attest that this is our reality. Being torn, constantly, back and forth between family duties and selfish, egotistical, narcissistic (but only for women—in men, these are admirable, positive attributes) pursuits, including the seemingly innocuous writing of a personal journal. But it isn't just a gendered issue. It is also a racial and class issue.

Audre Lorde, African American poet and author of the powerful pathography, or story of her illness, *The Cancer Journals*, wrote this in her journal on April 6, 1980, six months post-mastectomy, "Somedays [sic], if bitterness were a whetstone, I could be sharp as grief." In the same month, she gave a speech at Amherst College in which she pointed out that prose, which includes most journal writing, requires "a room of one's own" and "reams of paper" and "plenty of time." She makes the case for why so many marginalized people write poetry instead of prose: because, she contends, poetry is the most economical, and can be done between shifts, "in the hospital pantry, on the subway, and on scraps of paper." It strikes me that poetry may also be the safest form of writing for many people, what with its oftentimes oblique and veiled references.

This reminds me of the many times in my life that, while working in busy clinics, I escaped to bathroom stalls and scribbled down thoughts, feelings, reflections, and insights that I would later—in the privacy of my own room and journal—incorporate into more complete prose. Recording existence. My existence. My resistance. I'd write on scraps of paper, blank patient chart notepaper, paper towels, paper napkins, even—a few times in desperation—toilet paper. More recently, while visiting my elderly father, who was slowly dying of congestive heart failure, I stood in the basement of his home pretending to be busy doing his laundry, but instead slumped against a heavily cobwebbed table, writing on the blank side of an empty cardboard box of dryer sheets. "I can't believe I'm back here. I have to get away—and soon—or I will go stark raving mad."

Reading back through my journals, I notice how often I've lamented the lack of time and space in which to write—to be a writer—and times when I recognized the irony: that I was writing so many words, so many journal entries, about not being a writer. But I've always wondered: what makes anyone a writer, a real writer? Is it someone who makes a living from writing, or who is supported by someone else's career or inheritance while they spend their days writing? Is it someone who has published written work in a journal or magazine? Is it someone who has published a book? Or is it someone who feels compelled to write, whose orientation to the world is primarily through the written word?

Terry Tempest Williams, in her book *When Women Were Birds: Fifty-Four Variations on Voice*, tells of receiving her mother's journals, left to her with the admonition that she was to read them only after her mother's death, which occurred from breast cancer at age fifty-four. Williams comes from a long line of Utah Mormon women whose religious duties as mothers include keeping journals of their lives. After her mother's death, Williams went to read these journals, and all of them—row upon bookshelf row of beautifully bound notebooks—were blank. She writes, "When I opened my mother's journals and read emptiness, it translated to longing, that same hunger and thirst Mother translated to me. I will rewrite this story, create my own story on the pages of my mother's journals." That rewriting became her book.

Our biological mothers are—always, and so much more so than our fathers—mysteries. We have swum in their oceanic seas and been attached to them through that cord of life that is never completely severed. After my own mother's death from breast cancer, over seven years ago now, I went in search of her. My mother was a professional artist, so I knew to look for her first in her art studio.

She was there on her paint-splattered blue wooden stool. She was there in the piles of collographs, etchings, watercolors, and oil paintings. She was there in all her little sketch notebooks, in one of which she had written on the first page: "Christmas, 1965. Sanibel Island. A time to begin again. A time of renewal." I find it significant that this was the year that I—her youngest, and somewhat of a surprise child—had started kindergarten, freeing her time for artwork. She was there in her medical diary: notations on medications, chemo treatments, side effects, diagnoses, mixed in with notes about letters she'd written and how many loads of laundry she had done. January 28, 2008, the year of her death: "Definitely in remission." Whenever she refers to herself, it is with the third-person first initial "R."

Intrigued, yet disappointed, by the clues to my mother I'd unearthed in her studio, I returned to that cobwebbed basement of my parents' house, where in a corner beside the laundry area I discovered a battered old black steamer trunk, covered with faded European hotel stickers such as the one for the Grand Hotel Heidelberg. Opening it, I found a cache of my mother's past: A copy of her birth certificate from Tokyo, Japan, from April 1923—the year the Great Kanto Earthquake and ensuing dragon twist fire destroyed so much in its path. Crumbling photo albums full of black-and-white photos from my mother's childhood through her college years. Handmade cloth dolls. Sketch pads full of watercolor and charcoal drawings from her art school days. Letters to her written by Jack, her fiancé who was killed in the Normandy invasion. Angst-filled poetry she wrote the summer she learned of his death. A roll of creamed-white silk from Japan, the silk torn and stained brown in a few places.

And in this steamer trunk I found her fifty-page, handwritten memoir—a memoir she had never mentioned to me—in a lovely gilt-edged notebook, with this opening entry:

Sanibel Island, January 5, 1990. Now, with retirement official for us, it seems fitting to begin a journal reflecting remembrances of past years, something I wish my own parents and grandparents had done in their time. Family histories weren't all that important to me in my younger days but, with the passing of earlier generations, I realize how much of human experience has been lost to me and my children that can no longer be retrieved.

Her closing sentence in her memoir comes after describing finishing her master of fine arts degree from Temple University: "I was considering a career in teaching at the time but somehow John [my father] intervened and we married in September, on the 13th, 1947!" Gaps. Silences. My mother ends her memoir with her marriage and an exclamation point.

I found no other memoirs or journals written by my mother, but in this trunk she had carefully stored a torn portion of my maternal great-grandmother's journal, as well as a travel journal written by my maternal great-aunt Annie. This travel journal, handwritten in a composition notebook the summer of 1931, recorded Great-Aunt Annie's solo tour of Europe, sailing on the TSS *Rotterdam* from New York and then traveling by rail and boat through the Netherlands, Germany, Austria, Switzerland, France, Belgium, and on to London before returning to her Philadelphia home and job as a secretary. She reports that she ate too much throughout the trip, her clothes becoming tighter. She records historical facts about all the cities visited, and her impressions of art in galleries. Conversations with various men she met along the way. She becomes acutely homesick while staying at the Grand Hotel Heidelberg, precipitated by a seemingly trivial experience trying to buy postage stamps. Even within the dry recitation—of facts, places visited, famous statues and buildings and paintings seen, meals eaten, snatches of conversations—her distinct silhouette can be discerned.

Now, piecing together entries in my mother's memoir with this travel journal, I discover that in 1931, my great-aunt Annie had turned thirty-six, had never been married, and had just recovered from a complete hysterectomy to remove uterine fibroids—a procedure in which her surgeons decided she no longer needed her vagina, so they simply sewed it shut. When she married my great-uncle Aaron when she was fifty, she had to have her vagina unsewn. This context makes my rereading of her travel journal so much more interesting. Monday July 6, 1931, Lady's Night dance on the boat the second day into her European trip: "Stayed up until almost one o'clock. All right for one night but I do not see enough in it. Such an artificial life."

What is not said can bellow in our ears once we begin to listen, to pay attention. I have learned to pay attention to the silences, the gaps in my own life. I note the times when I stopped writing in my journal. Like after my own first marriage at age twenty-two, when I wrote, "I am so happy that I do not need to write in my journal." I heeded too readily—in my then Christian fervor—C. S. Lewis's admonition that journal writing was a drug, an addiction leading only to wallowing in suffering and sinful self-absorption.

I note the times when I did write in my journal but was aware, at the time, that what I was writing was not the whole truth. Not that I was lying so much as purposefully not admitting to myself—to my journal as myself—what was going on emotionally in my life. Frissons: those shivers of recognition of omission of something vitally important. Shivers: the body recognizing cold and strong emotion. Frissons are the auroras, the signals of pivotal moments; warnings, if not heeded, of a seizure ahead. I have learned to pay attention to the silences, the gaps, the frissons.

Friday, December 18, 2015. Seattle, Washington. 7:30 a.m. Rainy and dreary. I had a dream within a dream last night, where I discovered a hidden, closed-off, beautiful part of our house while I was repairing a rotten, disintegrating wall. And in my dream I remembered that I had dreamed of this before. What's that about? Parts of myself I am now discovering, dusting off, beginning to use?

What is it that compels some people, including me, to become writers of their lives, if not published authors? What does that say about them, about me? And what does that say about others who do not record their lives through words? Are they less "deep," or are they happier and more well-adjusted to life? Joan Didion, in her essay "On Keeping a Notebook," says of this compulsion, which she admits to having: "Keepers of private notebooks are a different breed altogether, lonely and resistant rearrangers of things, anxious malcontents, children afflicted apparently at birth with some presentiment of loss."

I am intrigued by the fact that so many journal writers, as well as so many published authors, such as Virginia Woolf, believe that nothing has really happened until it has been described, until it has been written down. "From the beginning, I knew the diary wasn't working, but I couldn't stop writing. I couldn't think of any other way to avoid getting lost in time," writes Sarah Manguso in her book *Ongoingness: The End of a Diary*. At a personal level, does this signify a fractured self with a tenuous hold on reality?

Perhaps the journal documents the existence and survival of the self. As Joyce Carol Oates states about Thoreau after she read his journals, "he is the most acute of observers of nature and of human nature; an analyst of his 'self' in the Whitmanesque sense, the 'self' that is all selves, the transcendent universal." And, in the introduction to her own published journals, Oates asks:

> Is the keeping of a journal primarily providing solace to the self, through a "speaking" voice that is one's own voice subtly transformed? A way of dispelling loneliness, a way of comfort? . . . It might be argued that, like our fingerprints and voice "prints," our journal-selves are distinctly our

own; try as we might, we can't elude them; the person one is, is evident in every line; not a syllable can be falsified.

Stories that people tell about their life experiences, including the stories within journal entries, are the building blocks of identity. As narrative goes, writing is an important process of self-construction, of figuring out the self in relation to others and to the world. The development of the self is always in relation to the Other, something which most journal-writing includes in spades—especially early in life: parents, siblings, teachers, peers, moving on to intimate partners, co-workers, neighbors. Life with all these Others. And then, throughout life, finding ways to bring in, to integrate, painful experiences into our life stories, to find some sort of agency so that the traumas are not just something that happened to us, they are something that—both good and bad—become part of who we are. Writing about important life events is a way to author the self.

Journal writing is a lifeline umbilical cord nourishing and protecting the always-developing self, especially when that self is under extreme duress, such as the long line of people imprisoned, kept in solitary confinement, who maintained a link to sanity, a tether to the self, through writing, recording, scratching on prison walls, composing in the mind when denied actual writing implements. People who managed to maintain an intact selfhood through writing, through narration.

Journal entries are by their nature episodic, no matter how much time a person spends writing. They are fragments, scraps of stories, of an individual's life story. The journals become artifacts of memory, artifacts of a life.

I reflect on the various uses of my journals and of my journal writing that I've experienced so far in my life. Recording secret confidences with my dragon protector. Venting righteous indignation towards parents, teachers, co-workers, lovers. Rereading all my journals as a young adult in nursing school, looking for clues to my development of and then slow recovery from anorexia. (I thought I could write a scholarly paper using this as case study material.)

My journals as sources of remembrance of what I was thinking and feeling at certain times in my life: Reading back over my journals and reflecting on who I'd been then, and the changes and insights I'd had at certain points. Looking at how I described the depths of my depression while in the pit of despair.

My journals as primary source material: Researching and writing my medical memoir, *Catching Homelessness*. And, more recently, searching back through my journals for diagnostic symptoms of what was to become my mystery illness—my mixed connective tissue autoimmune disease.

Noticing the important gaps and silences and incoherent babbling discontinuities—what I did not write about, or at least did not write about clearly—at certain times, and why. My fractured selves stitched together lovingly by the thread of words—and by the thread of the silent absence of words.

This excerpt from Virginia Woolf's diary from Monday, January 20, 1919:

> I note however that this diary writing does not count as writing, since I have just re-read my year's diary and am much struck by the rapid hap-hazard gallop at which it swings along, sometimes indeed jerking almost intolerably over the cobbles. Still if it were not written rather faster than the fastest type-writing, if I stopped and took thought, it would never be written at all; and the advantage of this method is that it sweeps up accidentally several stray matters which I should exclude if I hesitated, but which are diamonds in the dustheap. If Virginia Woolf at the age of 50, when she sits down to build her memoirs out of these books, is unable to make a phrase as it should be made, I can only condole with her and remind her of the existence of the fireplace, where she has my leave to burn these pages to so many black films with red eyes in them. But how I envy her the task I am preparing for her! There is none I should like better. Already my 37th birthday next Saturday is robbed of some of its terrors by the thought.

According to the Virginia Woolf scholar, Louise DeSalvo, twenty years after she wrote this diary entry, Virginia Woolf consulted her early journals when she wrote her memoir piece, "A Sketch of the Past." This was in the spring of 1939, at age fifty-seven, and just two years before her death. From Woolf's diary entry from April 15, 1939: "I'm interested in depression, & make myself play a game of assembling the fractured pieces."

I compare my sources and find it intriguing that this sentence was deleted from the heavily edited version that Woolf's husband, Leonard, used for what he published for her as *A Writer's Diary*. Why did he delete this sentence? Did he somehow want to keep the focus of the book away from her bouts of depression, from what led to her eventual death by drowning?

In addition, DeSalvo points out that although there is ample evidence that Virginia Woolf spoke with her sister and her husband about her history of childhood sexual abuse by her older half-brother, "A Sketch of the Past" is the first—and only—time she was to write of his abuse. She makes no mention of it in her diary—something that people have tried to use as evidence that the abuse never happened. What is more likely is that when the fifty-seven-year-old Virginia Woolf sat down to reread her journals in order to write her memoirs, in order to understand her depression, she recognized the frissons, the gaps, the silences within her earlier diaries. She found a way to assemble the fractured pieces.

Saturday, December 19, 2015. Seattle, Washington. 8:00 a.m. For the essay I'm writing on journal writing, I need to go through my collection of journals. But that's not something I want to do with a house full of people. I need space and privacy for that endeavor.

Concerns for privacy always surround the practice of personal journal writing. That concern starts early, with diaries for young people—especially for girls—often made with locks and small keys, the better to protect from the prying eyes of parents and siblings. Anaïs Nin, whose main writing was her journals, kept a journal from age eleven into her seventies, and stored them in a bank vault—except, of course, for the volumes she had published. Beatrix Potter, who lived with strict Victorian parents, devised a code when she was nine that she used to write her journals—a code so complex it took cryptologists years to decipher it after her death.

Christina Baldwin, who teaches journal writing, encourages her students to write some sort of admonishment at the front of their journals, stating that it is private, not meant to be read by anyone without permission from the author of the journal. In her book *One to One: Self-Understanding through Journal Writing*, she reports that her students have hidden their journals in cookbooks, in suitcases or briefcases, in the trunk of a car. Then there is the reverse psychology practice of leaving personal journals out—not in-your-face aggressively out, but just out in plain sight so that they appear something routine, and boring perhaps: there they are on our bookshelves among all the other books gathering dust. The more we try to protect, hide, and hold private, the greater the propensity for the curious to want to discover, to pry open. As Baldwin reminds us, "We are paranoid about privacy, because we know that we have impulses to invade the privacy of others."

At some point, typically as we grow older and have accumulated a cache of journals, as I have, it is important to face the question of what we want done with our journals, how to document our wishes, and who we trust to carry out our wishes. Include our journals in our wills, and update as needed. Name an executor. Although history bears out that our wishes on such matters—no matter how meticulous our planning—are often not followed.

In a fascinating and slightly macabre article in the *Paris Review*, "Books and Bodies: On Organs and Literary Estates," Casey N. Cep writes:

> Organ donation provides an apt analogy for posthumous publishing, which presumes to take into account the wishes of dead authors, but involves a similarly complex set of actors. . . . When it comes to organ donations, the wishes of the deceased are only one part of the complicated matrix that determines whether organs are actually harvested. The same is true for authors who leave behind work, finished or unfinished, public or private. Books, like bodies, are not always the property of their originators.

Cep is, of course, here referring to authors who were published before their deaths. These same principles, though, apply to public figures who are not authors, as well as to private individuals.

There are the famous examples of next-of-kin and other executors who did not follow the wishes of the deceased. Franz Kafka, who left his literary estate to his friend and fellow writer Max Brod, asked that all his work be burned unread. Instead, Brod published Kafka's literary works posthumously, arguing that he had told Kafka he would not destroy them and Kafka left them to him anyway. Virgil asked that *The Aeneid* be incinerated after his death. Virginia Woolf ended her suicide note to her husband with the words, "Would you destroy all my papers." Fortunately for us, he did not do this. Writing about this topic in the *Telegraph*, Nicolette Jones states, "Burned manuscripts are a death on top of death, which is why so many people are tempted into the morally debatable position of ignoring the wishes of authors who want their writings destroyed."

After Sylvia Plath gassed herself to death while her two young children slept—protected by Plath—in a room nearby, her estranged husband, the poet Ted Hughes, inherited—along with her alma mater, Smith College—all her unpublished work, including her journals. From Hughes's foreword to the edited version of *The Journals of Sylvia Plath*:

> Two more notebooks survived for a while, maroon-backed ledgers like the '57–'59 volume, and it continued the record from late '59 to within three days of her death [in February 1963]. The last of these contained entries for several months, and I destroyed it because I did not want her children to have to read it (in those days I regarded forgetfulness as an essential part of survival). The other disappeared.

In a note he includes later in the book, he reports that Plath was rereading her early journals as source material when—in the spring and summer of 1961—she was working on her memoir, *The Bell Jar*. After Ted Hughes's death in 1998, Smith College released the unabridged version of Plath's journals, but the two journals Hughes says he either destroyed or "went missing" have never resurfaced.

In the seemingly never-ending tragedy of Plath's life, her son, Nicholas Hughes, an Alaskan marine biologist and potter, hung himself in March 2009. His sister said he'd been battling depression for some time. He was single and childless and only forty-seven years old when he died. Did he read his mother's unabridged journals, and if so, did this deepen his depression? This question haunts me, since depression reaches its hyphae up through my own family tree. I would not want my words—or my lack of words—in my journals to hurt my son.

While researching the topic of what people do with their journals and why, I posed the question on various social media sites. Answers came from people who had decided to burn all their journals, and they either "felt so much freer" or "regret it now, as I'd like to have them." A man living in a fire-prone area of the West said he stored his journals in a plastic bin in the back of his pickup truck and drove them around whenever he needed to evacuate. Another person said she wrote journal pages and tore them into fragments, which she then stored in an antique suitcase, later pulling ones out at random to incorporate into her poetry. And, in a *New York Times Style Magazine*, the novelist Heidi Julavits writes of having met an Italian artist who encases books in white plaster:

> He provided this service to an Italian aristocrat, a married woman who'd had the same lover for decades and who'd kept a diary of their affair. Now in her 60s, she did not want to risk anyone reading her diary, nor did she want to burn or throw it away. She asked the artist to turn it into an innocuous-seeming sculpture. She displays the plaster diary in her house.

I wonder if, after her death, someone will decide to chip away the white plaster and read her words.

Sunday, December 20, 2015. Seattle, Washington. 9:00 a.m. I got a lot of writing done this morning, plowing along on my "An Over-Examined Life" essay. I am now writing in my journal about writing about journal writing. Is that meta-journaling or meta-meta-journaling?

When does this journal writing endeavor become not just an examined (healthy) but an overexamined (obsessive-compulsive/unhealthy) life? How do you know when you're tipping yourself out through the therapeutic window and falling into the Slough of Despond?

The health benefits—and detriments—of writing a journal, or more specifically, of writing through traumas and troublesome parts of our lives, are beginning to be understood. One of the leading experts in this area, James W. Pennebaker, contends that mounting research evidence attests to the multiple positive health effects of writing about and through trauma, but mainly if the writing is a mixture of emotions and cognitive "thinking through" the facts, and if both positive and negative consequences of traumatic events are addressed. Not surprisingly—at least for those of us who have spent time wallowing in negative emotions and memories—excessive rumination, writing over and over again about the same troubling event, is neither helpful nor healthful. Finding some way out of that wallowing, being able to step back, to gain some emotional distance from this sort of stuttering, incoherent rant, is something we all have to find our way to, whether on our own, through wake-up calls from loved ones, or through professional therapy.

As an example of what is perhaps a different sort of overexamined life, I am reminded of Robert Shields, a Protestant minister and English teacher who lived with his wife in the small town of Dayton, in southeastern Washington State. Shields wrote (typed, to be exact) in his diary for four hours a day, recording his life—what he ate, what he bought and how much it cost, his bowel and bladder habits, his dreams, his spiritual beliefs—in five-minute increments. He pasted his typed diary entries into a logbook, along with taped oddities such as soup can labels, dead spiders, nail clippings, and nose hairs. He did this for over twenty-five years, until a stroke kept him from being able to type for the last decade of his life and his wife refused to take his diary dictation.

When Shields died, in 2007 at age eighty-nine, he had a 37.5 million-word diary—ninety-four boxes of diaries, which he had arranged to donate to Washington State University, even giving the university $75,000 for archiving his collection. In a 1994 *Seattle Times* article by Kit Boss, Shields admitted to no longer traveling because it disrupted his diary-writing. He hoped his diary collection would be of use to future historians, psychologists, and sociologists. His twin daughters, one a lawyer and the other a physician, entreat the reporter to quote them as both leading "normal lives."

I tend to agree with their assessment of their father's overexamined life, because his journal writing seems in excess: journal writing wasn't enriching his life but rather was getting in the way of his living a full life. But did he recognize this as a problem? I suppose we will have to wait the fifty years he stipulated for his journal collection to be sealed, before we know the answer to that question.

But, perhaps Shields was right. Perhaps at some point in the future, people will find a positive use for his voluminous personal records. Henry David Thoreau's journals, with their meticulous recordings, not only of his inner musings on his self, include detailed accounts of weather, temperature, rainfall, the exact blooming times of plants in the immediate vicinity of his home in Concord, Massachusetts. As Andrea Wulf reports in her April 19, 2013, *New York Times* article "A Man for All Seasons," the Boston University professor of biology Richard Primack, and colleagues at Harvard, are using Thoreau's journals to help document the effects of climate change.

I fear I may be overexamining this topic, because I grow paranoid. While doing research for this article, I stumble upon a Free Books table outside the health sciences library that contains a gorgeous hand-bound journal, covered with handmade paper and with an attached bookmark in the shape of an oak leaf. It is so surprisingly beautiful sitting there in an otherwise tasteless, soulless, functional environment. Like a shiny jewel: irresistible. Having brought it home, I'm now suspicious that it contains some secret electronic tracking device and that I've unwittingly become part of some student's research study—on journal writing.

Sunday, January 17, 2016. Seattle, Washington. 6:00 a.m. Raining. I'm waiting for the coffee to kick in so I can write. As in really write—work on my journal writing essay which I've made a lot of progress on. I think I found a good structure for it—using brief quotes from my journal entries—from this journal no less.

As I wrote the above journal entry in my composition notebook, my favorite pen, a Pilot Precise V5 Rolling Ball Stick Pen Extra Fine, ran out of ink. Grabbing a new one to continue writing, I discovered that it began to bleed and blotch all over the page of my journal. Frustrated, I changed to a cheap ballpoint pen. I had just been reading the unabridged journals of Virginia Woolf, where she recorded similar frustrations with various pens, finally settling on one she liked. Saturday, April 17, 1897, she wrote, "I shall not again desert my beloved Swan [pen]."

I spend time researching the Swan pen's history, origin, and fan pages. Dismayed by the fact that Swan pens are no longer made, I consider purchasing an antique one to see what writing with it is like—to see what was so special about this pen that caused Virginia Woolf to love it so. But an antique Swan pen, as well as the ivory-leafed pocket notebook I could buy from the store in Indiana, remain unpurchased. I do not want to accumulate more detritus to have to deal with. I am trying to rid my life of detritus.

During his recent holiday break from work, my partner, Peter, decided to clean out the garage in preparation for us moving house someday relatively soon—a future house that we will jointly own. I am not as excited about this prospect as is Peter. There are so many buried truths in my house and in my garden that I do not want to leave behind.

Peter walked into my office one morning soon after Christmas, as I was, of course, writing in my journal. He carried two cardboard boxes he had just unearthed in the garage—boxes that contained some of my old, forgotten belongings. Old photographs and letters, my high school diploma, my original first marriage license—and, as I dug through the musty boxes, two additional journals of mine. Not the lost journal I sought, but more recent travel journals. So, I added them to the growing collection of journals—journals which now seem to mate and reproduce themselves in dark, musty corners, as do the mice and rats we've found evidence of in our garage.

There they are, laid out once more on the floor of my office at home, my collection of 123 journals:

- Seven journals from my childhood, starting when I was twelve: "Thursday the 22nd of February 1973 just wasn't my day. Two people I know went to the office and I lost a boyfriend. Oh well, didn't and don't (more than ever) care for boyfriends." Journals I made myself from materials in my mother's studio. One is covered with blue turtle stamp markings, the stamp I carved from an India ink gum eraser. Then I graduated to using spiral notebooks through my high school years. During my childhood through high school I averaged writing 30 journal pages a year.

- Two journals from my Oberlin College years. Spiral-bound notebooks like the ones I used for class note-taking. An average of sixty-six journal pages a year.

- Seven journals from after my college graduation through the years of my return to living in Richmond, Virginia. Mostly spiral-bound notebooks, switching to black-and-white composition notebooks my last few years in Richmond. The switch came when I had blank pages left in my organic chemistry lab notebook and had no money to buy another. I continued to write only on the right-hand side of the pages. During this time span I averaged seventy pages a year.

- Twelve journals from my Baltimore years. I continued to write in composition notebooks, but towards the end, I switched to writing on the right-hand pages first and then returning by writing on the left-hand pages. I averaged 328 pages a year.

- Ninety-five journals so far of my Seattle years. Most of these journals are composition notebooks, with a few smaller spiral-bound travel journals, such as the notebook I used on a hike along the

Pacific Coast with my then boyfriend—where I documented the precise moment of our demise as a couple. I have averaged 881 pages per year.

- In 2015, I wrote a total of 1,082 pages, confirming my suspicion that my journal-writing velocity has increased. This is something I find ironic, since I've also become a "real" (published) writer of more than academic journal articles during this time span. As of December 31, 2015, I have an estimated 21,873 pages of handwritten journal entries. I shudder to contemplate how many more I will write during my lifetime.

What to do with them? Do I throw them out, recycle them, or burn them in a huge bonfire—a bonfire of the vanities—reduce them "to so many black films with red eyes in them," as Virginia Woolf phrased it? Do I continue writing my journals as long as I am a sentient being—squirreling them away somewhere safe—and then let whoever is in charge of disposition of my remains—my organs, my journals—decide what to do with them? Do I seek out a women's studies department or a university archive to donate them to, as if I or what I've written matter to anyone in the future? Do I let my son decide what to do with them? Do I want him to read my journals? Do I—as my son the practical historian recommends—scan them into one long digital file and store them ... where? On some virtual journal cloud?

My son knows I am researching and writing this essay. One recent evening at the dinner table, he asks, "So, what do you want me to do with all your journals?" I tell him I'm still searching for the answer and I'll let him know once I've figured it out.

But for now, I have at least found a suitable repository for my collection of journals. From the family of a recently deceased neighbor, I bought a lovely Taiwanese rosewood chest with a fierce dragon carved on the front. Situated in a corner of my home office next to Great-Aunt Annie's steamer trunk, this chest is now filled with my journals, a few spare blankets, and the stained Japanese silk from my mother. Kwan Yin, the goddess of compassion, came with the chest, so she stands guard over them all. It has become my "Dear Dragon" rosewood journal chest.

My journals document my travels and my survival; they are like my old umbilical cord, connecting me to all my former selves. For now, they will accompany me wherever I go. They—even more so than my current home and garden—contain the half-buried truths I want to remember. If home is where I am known and where I come to know myself, my journals are my "castle out of pebbles," my carapace—they are home.

Fourteen

Lab Notebook

Tell me, what is it you plan to do
with your one wild and precious life?
—Mary Oliver

Item: Spiral-bound notebook, nine and a half by six inches, college ruled, 102 sheets, with a green marbled cover. On the front is the name, B. J. Ensign, written in blue ink, a red-construction-paper nonanatomical heart glued below the name, with a partially torn gold-foil smaller heart glued inside the red heart. And the word *disguise* written below the heart. The sale price of the notebook, one dollar eighty-nine cents, is written in pencil in the top right corner. Inside, there are three sections separated by plastic tabs: (1) a red tab for Vertebrate Physiology Lab Notes, (2) a yellow tab for Psychophysiology of Religion, and (3) a blue tab for C. S. Lewis.

The Psychophysiology of Religion and C. S. Lewis courses were both private readings I took with professors of religion at Oberlin College. I was a biology and religion double major, and this notebook is from 1980, spring semester of my freshman year. I was nineteen years old. Oberlin offered religion as a humanistic discipline rather than as a theological undertaking. I was drawn to the intersection of objective science and subjective religion—I wanted to pause in that space.

Warren F. Walker, professor of anatomy and physiology, was my academic advisor. His field of research was the anatomy and physiology of locomotion, and especially of turtle locomotion. His wife, Tilly, told me that he had studied their children as they learned to crawl and then walk. He and his wife were members of First Church in Oberlin, United Church of Christ, and they invited me to join them there for services. I went on most Sundays, mainly for the music, since the church drew from the talented students in the Oberlin Conservatory of Music.

From my observations, Professor Walker kept science and religion in separate spheres. He had a notoriously bad sense of direction, a fact I found surprising. When I worked as a lab assistant in one of his courses, I accompanied him on trips to an open market in Cleveland to buy lab animals (turtles, as I remember). He had a large round compass attached to his car dashboard, a compass which he consulted while driving the back roads between Oberlin and Cleveland. I assume he was unaware of the fact that such a compass is thrown off by its proximity to the car's engine and metal chassis.

These memories return to me as I read through my college lab notebook and personal journal from that time. I search for traces of my early exploration of the relationship between science and religion in my own life—and of where that quest has led me almost four decades later.

Lab Experiment #1, February 7, 1980
Vertebrate Physiology
Notes: Gastrocnemius Muscle Preparation. Five to ten minutes to anesthetize the frog; don't ever put H2O inside the animal—will destroy! Here is a diagram of the Harvard inductorium with a battery at one end and stimulating electrodes at the other end. Practice with finger and tongue using the stimulator. Set up smoked drum sheet (kymograph) to record waves. Dissect out gastrocnemius muscle from anesthetized frog and attach it to the inductorium. Record the electrical wave responses to a set of increasing volts and durations of the stimuli.

Psychophysiology of Religion
According to Robert E. Ornstein in *The Psychology of Consciousness*, there is a duality of human nature: (1) analytical, logical, reasoning; and (2) intuitive, imaginative, creative. Right and left hemispheres of the brain exist with separate functions in split-brain experiments. There are increased alpha-waves in meditative states. Using EEGs, there are longer waves associated with sleep or deep relaxation. There is an inability to verbalize mystical experiences, perhaps because insights from the right hemisphere might not

fit into sequential left hemisphere terms.

C. S. Lewis

In the afterword of *A Grief Observed*, Chad Walsh writes of the blue hills on the horizon near C. S. Lewis's childhood home—distant hills that symbolized for Lewis the unknown, the numinous, or what he later came to call "Joy" or "Romance," a hunger for something else that was what drew him to Christianity.

I remember feeling disappointed—and somehow duped—when I realized that my beloved childhood Narnia series by Lewis was really a magic-wardrobe sleight-of-hand magic trick of a Sunday school lesson. As a child, I did not like King of the Jungle male lion Aslan and could not understand why the personification of evil was cast as Jadis, the White Witch. Jadis, who was protected by a host of fierce beings, including a Minotaur and hags. Jadis, who knew how to use the Deplorable Word, who had caused the land of Narnia to be in perpetual winter—like the nuclear winter we were taught about in school as we did drills ducking under our desks. Which also did not make any sense to me. How would huddling under the gum-encrusted wooden desks possibly protect us from the fallout of the Deplorable Word? And how could one word contain so much power?

Lab Experiment #2, February 14, 1980
Vertebrate Physiology

Notes: Redo the kymograph from last week and this time, Do It Right! Stimulus, signal magnet, tuning fork: start turning the drum, then start the tuning fork, then stimulate the muscle, and calculate the velocity of shortening, the velocity of the muscle contraction. Need to know latent time, the time between stimulus and response. Remember: Velocity = Distance/Time.

Psychophysiology of Religion

Continuing to read *The Psychology of Consciousness* by Ornstein, I note where he quotes the psychiatrist Arthur J. Deikman as stating, "Ordinary language is structured to follow the logical development of one idea at a time, and it may be quite inadequate to express an experience encompassing a large number of concepts simultaneously."

C. S. Lewis

In *The Pilgrim's Regress* I note on page 169 where Lewis asserts that the world is a great imagination of one mind in which we live. Lewis develops his contention of reason as the organ of truth versus imagination as the organ of meaning. It strikes me that the word organ is an odd one here. Lewis is using it in the *Oxford English Dictionary* now-marked-as-obsolete sense of "a mental or spiritual faculty regarded as an instrument of the mind or soul." I find that I, the now fifty-six-year-old formerly BJ currently Josephine, consult the *Oxford English Dictionary* frequently in all matters of direction, of where our words—my words—come from and where they lead.

Lab Experiment #3, February 21, 1980
Vertebrate Physiology

Notes: Do experiment #3 even if not finished with #s 1 and 2. There are three parts to this experiment: (1) divide into groups of four students and use one frog per group; (2) each student does his or her own summation of response; and, (3) finish by doing the Saient Georgi experiment with a glycerinated frog muscle strip, adding (in order) ATP, potassium chloride and magnesium chloride salts, and EGTA (ethylene glycol tetraacetic acid). Results: nothing happened because the muscle died!

Psychophysiology of Religion

Why are we drawn to mystical experiences? Arthur Deikman contends it is perhaps because most of our current problems center on the need for a shift towards a consciousness of the interconnectedness of life and away from the survival of the individual.

C. S. Lewis

In my private reading professor Gilbert C. Meilaender's book *The Taste for the Other: The Social and Ethical Thought of C. S. Lewis*, I note his highlighting of the fact that in Lewis's fantasy book *Till We Have Faces*, the female protagonist Orual had to be taught a lesson in independence: she had to be broken before she could "have a face," before she could be reborn. I also note that the purported model for the character Orual was Lewis's wife, Joy, who died of cancer soon after their marriage. I wonder what a feminist critique of this would be, but decide that Professor Meilaender is not the sort of person with whom to raise this question.

Lab Experiment #4, February 28, 1980
Vertebrate Physiology

Part A: Kymograph with isometric levers. Use sartorius muscle. Bone attached to each end. Put glass probe under tendon attaching sartorius to knee, tear the fascia working upwards. *Use two muscles together, the sartorius and adductor magnus, as this is safer, less likely to injure. Remember: Work = Force x Distance.

Part B: Get isotonic information from other groups. Expand axis to half a page. Label graph and axis. Draw smooth line through the graph.

Psychophysiology of Religion

I read of the importance of the role of myth in our lives, myth as unconscious storytelling. And of the fact that biofeedback is the synthesis of analytical (objective, scientific) and holistic (subjective) states. Biofeedback uses electronic monitoring of stress-related states as biological feedback to the person, helping him or her learn to modulate stress through meditation and other techniques.

C. S. Lewis

Lewis claims that myth does not refer to the (non)historical, but rather to the (non)describable. Are *(non)historical* and *(non)describable* even words? Shouldn't they be *ahistorical* and *indescribable*, but then, if they are these words, are these words similarly comparable to (non)describable and (non) historical?

In my journal I write that my head hurts from reading C. S. Lewis and asking myself these sorts of questions. Perhaps I would benefit from biofeedback? I have developed migraines, an annoying heart arrhythmia, and times of profound depression, lamenting in my journal, "So many damn anxieties, hopes, fears, wants, dislikes. How can a mind think and feel so many different things at one time? I envision my head sparking, smoking, and finally blowing up under the strain of it all." I shut my notebook and go for a run in the city's graveyard.

Lab Experiment #5, March 6, 1980
Vertebrate Physiology

Nerves: Know the historical significance of this experiment and practice the proper handling of nerves. The first part is Galvani's experiment where he misinterpreted his data: the direct current due to metals he thought was electricity originating within the animal. First, pith the frog. Second, remove the abdominal viscera and locate the sciatic nerve along the back. Third, slip bar under plexus on both sides. The only contact with the nerves is with the copper bar. Fourth, touch the leg with the iron bar and watch what happens. Results: The frog jumped.

Then, do the second experiment of the action-current, rheoscopic frog, laying a cut frog gastrocnemius muscle with nerve attached across the frog's beating heart, and watch what happens. Results: The leg muscle contracted in rhythm with the beating heart.

Psychophysiology of Religion

Carl Sagan, in *The Dragons of Eden*, writes that split-brain function studies indicate that the corpus callosum is such a complex structure that it must mean that interaction between the two hemispheres is a vital human function. Significantly, in drug-induced and in dream states, there is often a "watcher," and one side of the brain (or "self") asks the watcher, "Who are you?" and the watcher replies, "Who wants to know?" This is similar to Sufi questions.

C. S. Lewis

In his autobiography, *Surprised by Joy: The Shape of My Early Life*, Lewis writes of his parents. His father was Irish of Welsh descent, with a quick and fierce temper and very much ruled by emotions, while his mother had an aristocratic, proper British background. Lewis was closest to his cool, collected, intellectual mother, and this caused him to distrust all emotions until much later in life when he fell in love with a woman named Joy.

I think of how different my own parents are from each other—and from me, as I struggle to discover who I am. My father's capricious anger and strange spasms of inappropriate shows of affection that leave me bewildered and disoriented. The fact that he is a Presbyterian minister. My mother's cool, detached, intellectual, darkly creative approach to life.

I was closest to my mother, but that left me profoundly confused since she refused to believe or protect me from my father. Besides migraines, a heart arrhythmia, and depression, I developed panic attacks, except I did not have that name for them. Instead, upon reading the work of Saint John of the Cross, I called them dark nights of the soul, and fervently prayed for healing. Prayer, for me, did not work, and I continued to have many dark nights of the soul.

Lab Experiment #6, March 13, 1980
Vertebrate Physiology

Notes: Nerve conduction tests extend into refractory period, action potential, summation of excitation, and conduction frequency, using the oscilloscope and the electrode chamber. Preparation of nerve: (1) decapitate the frog; (2) pith the spinal cord; (3) dissect out the sciatic nerve as per last week's instructions; (4) cut nerve off between where it emerges from the spinal column and where it inserts onto the knee; and, (5) only use glass, not metal, and place the nerve in a bath of frog Ringer's solution in petri dish between experiments.

Psychophysiology of Religion

Carl Sagan writes of the myth of Prometheus (whose name is Greek for "foresight"), who was chained to a rock and had his liver continuously eaten by an eagle (Sagan says it was a vulture) in punishment by the gods for introducing culture, in the form of fire, to humans. Sagan points out that the modern science of electricity has its origins in the Italian anatomist Luigi Galvani and his "eighteenth-century experiments on the electrical stimulation of twitches of frogs." Sagan goes on to add that only a few decades later, Mary Wollstonecraft Shelley penned the tale of Dr. Frankenstein's monster brought to life by electrical currents.

Sagan asserts that what makes us distinctly human is our intelligence. As proof, he lists out brain to body mass ratios of various lower and higher animals, with humans being the highest. He does acknowledge that his argument breaks down when it comes to ants, decidedly lower animals, who have an astonishingly high brain to body mass ratio.

C. S. Lewis

Lewis admits to a lifelong phobia of insects that emerged during his childhood. In *Surprised by Joy* he writes, "You may add that in the hive and the anthill we see fully realized the two things that some of us dread most for our own species—the dominance of the female and the dominance of the collective." I record and highlight in yellow this quote in my notebook. Again, I wonder what feminist scholars would say about this, but I keep my thoughts to myself—and to my notebook. I am beginning to find C. S. Lewis's writings tiresome.

Lab Experiment #7, March 20, 1980

Vertebrate Physiology

Notes: (1) Pith a frog and place in clamp. Observe. Results: Frog became limp and even its abdomen sucked in with a loss of muscle tone at 2:15 minutes. (2) Apply 30 percent acetic acid solution to frog's inner thigh. Observe. Results: Large reaction with both legs moving, but delayed response (latent period) of 2 seconds. (3) Apply filter paper to frog's back. Observe. Results: Stronger reaction with frog jumping out of clamp and also moved its arms. (4) Tie one leg of frog with a tight ligature. Inject curare, then strychnine, apply electrical stimulation to sciatic nerve. Observe. Results: [A recording of these results is missing from my lab notebook.]

Psychophysiology of Religion

The human realization of the linear movement of time led to both fear and religion. From Robert S. Ellwood Jr.'s book *Religious and Spiritual Groups in Modern America*, I learn there are two basic types of religions in the world: (1) those grounded in cosmic wonder and communicated by exemplary personalities, and (2) those grounded in revelation within history and emissary communication of the revelation. Mysticism has been weeded out of Judeo-Christian forms of theology. Modern religious cults in the United States represent the exemplary form of religious life, with something—someone—tangible to worship and believe in. They are a reaction to the alienation of modern society, a reaction against science and technology.

C. S. Lewis

Lewis claims that the strongest argument for God lies in the near-universal experience of *sehnsucht*, "nostalgia": an underlying sense of displacement or alienation from what is desired, a numinous awareness of the uncanny and a dread of the power behind it. In *The Weight of Glory*, Lewis contends that if a man is hungry, it makes sense that he should have a stomach and be capable of eating.

But this analogy befuddled my nineteen-year-old self, especially given the fact that I was struggling with a profound eating disorder—anorexia—which I was perpetually trying to cure through prayer for a miracle from God—a God who I was unsure exists, or, if he/she/it exists, was for me. Again, I kept these doubts to myself, although I did write about them in my journal and in my lab notebook.

Lab Experiment #8, April 3, 1980
Vertebrate Physiology

Notes: Visual acuity is a measure of the smallest point where the human eye can discern two dots as two separate dots. Brighter light leads to better vision. The measure of dark adaptation for the human eye shows the important characteristic of sense organs in their ability to adapt. Most of the adaptation occurs in the sense receptors themselves, while some adaptation occurs in the brain. The sense organs vary in their ability for adaptation. Visual adapts a lot; light touch adapts very quickly; pressure adapts instantly. With lab partner, measure each other's visual acuity and adaptation using the adaptometer. Results: My lab partner Phil's visual acuity is 1.3 while my visual acuity is 1.5, meaning that we both have better than normal visual acuity. Using the adaptometer, Phil first saw the light after one minute; I first saw the light after thirty-five seconds.

Psychophysiology of Religion

While reading *The Psychology of Consciousness* by Robert E. Ornstein, I learn that the main alterations in our environment of which we might be aware are: (1) changes in light, including any seasonal variations in the length of day, and the biological rhythms associated with this, including menstrual cycles; (2) changes in the air around us, such as negative air ions from moving water (ocean waves, waterfalls, thunderstorms), which seem to have positive effects on our moods and overall health; and (3) gravity, which helps us with spatial awareness. Gestalt therapy is based on sensory awareness. One of the founders of this therapy, Frederick S. Perls, is quoted as stating its main maxim is "Lose your mind and come to your senses."

C. S. Lewis

Of his conversion to Christianity, Lewis writes, "I can never again believe that religion is manufactured out of our unconscious, starved desires and is a substitute for sex." He is, of course, here referring to the work of Sigmund Freud. But then I learn that Lewis likely had a long-standing, complex, if not outright-sexual relationship with a woman twenty-seven years his senior, a woman with whom he lived for more than three decades, a divorced mother of two children, an outspoken atheist, a woman he referred to as his mother. His biological mother died of cancer when he was a young boy. C. S. Lewis biographers surmise that this affair with Mrs. Janie Moore is what

Lewis referenced in his autobiography, *Surprised by Joy*, when he states he is purposefully omitting "one huge and complex episode." It seems Lewis did not have words to describe this core relationship.

Lab Experiment #9, April 10, 1980
Vertebrate Physiology
Notes: Heart electrical conduction tests using turtle (three-chambered) heart. Vagus experiment: (1) pull turtle's neck out; (2) cut hole in skin; (3) using blunt dissection, locate carotid arteries on each side of neck; (4) expose carotids by placing slip sleeve electrode under vagus nerve that runs along the carotid; and (5) press vagus nerve and observe. Results: Heart stops while vagus nerve is pressed.

Then, do production of heart block experiment, where heart block is the interference of the passage of electrical impulse from auricle to ventricle. (1) Put cord around auricles and draw up tightly, and (2) choke off auricular-ventricular junction and observe. Results: At certain pressure, heart block occurs, where the ventricle won't beat after the auricle beats.

Psychophysiology of Religion
William James, writing in *The Varieties of Religious Experience*, defines religion as "the feelings, acts and experiences of individual men in their solitude, so far as they apprehend themselves to stand in relation to whatever they may consider the divine." He also maintains that it doesn't work to explain religion in physical terms with an organic causation, such as saying that Saint Paul was an epileptic, pointing out that even scientific suppositions could be caused by a faulty liver.

C. S. Lewis
In *God in the Dock: Essays on Theology and Ethics*, Lewis writes of vivisection and asks if pain is an evil, answering the question in the affirmative, pointing out that it has to be because otherwise, why treat human pain? And therefore, isn't it evil to inflict pain on animals? He concludes with this statement: "The victory of vivisection marks a great advance in the triumph of ruthless, non-moral utilitarianism over the old world of ethical law; a triumph in which we, as well as animals, are already victims, and of which Dachau and Hiroshima mark the most recent achievements."

Reading this does not help my state of mind. In my journal I write, "I am in the midst of what can only be described as a deep, dark depression—pretty heavy, huh? I'm moody and bitchy. I'm also turning yellow. My hands, that is. I'm probably dying of some liver infection, so all these worries about the future are futile."

After this journal entry, I visit the student clinic and am told that my hands are turning yellow because I am eating too many carrots. This has to do with my eating disorder that as yet has gone undiagnosed or treated. But I attend a free food and feelings workshop in the college's counseling center. I sit in a circle with ten other young women while the older female therapist places one Ritz cracker on each of our tongues. She instructs us to close our mouths but not chew or swallow the cracker quite yet, and then leads us in a ten-minute guided meditation as the cracker dissolves in our mouths. And yes, I immediately make the connection with communion wafers, what with their alchemy, magic, transmutation, and my fervent prayers to be healed. My eating disorder continues unabated and unsatiated.

Lab Experiment #10, April 17, 1980
Vertebrate Physiology

Notes: Microcirculation experiments using a frog and then our own forearms. Using the microscope, observe and sketch the circulatory features of the web of the frog's foot, and then its lung. Note the presence and distribution of melanophores, pigment-containing cells. Apply two drugs, norepinephrine (vasoconstrictor) and ACh (vasodilator) to the lung and observe. Results: Norepinephrine did not affect lung circulation while ACH speeded up lung circulation. Rationale: The frog lung may not contain vasoconstrictor fibers.

Next, do the Forearm Triple Response test: Use edge of ruler to stroke length of own forearm vigorously ten times. Observe, record, and explain reaction. Results: (1) Red streak, or flare, caused by vasodilation where pain endings in skin give off branch to arterioles and cause arteriole dilation; (2) wheal or edema forms next partly due to release of histamine by damaged cells, which then causes the capillaries to leak fluid, hence, the swelling; and (3) white reaction caused by vasoconstriction.

Psychophysiology of Religion

"'Who—or what—am I?' seems to concern every inquiring mind in its own way. It is a question I most want answered and am least equipped by training to understand; the science I have learned is of objects, and no object is the self," states psychiatrist Arthur Deikman, in his essay "The Missing Center."

C. S. Lewis

There are such things as opulent melancholy and the idea of the quest that run throughout all writings of Lewis—an ongoing dialectic between joy and melancholy. Of note are the ambivalent properties of joy and the fact that C. S. Lewis said of joy that it has an object of desire, which to him was God, and that he experienced diminished joy after becoming a Christian. There is the underlying assumption that perhaps Lewis did not like being happy—that instead, he enjoyed being caught up in the compulsive search, the yearning, the *sehnsucht* nostalgia, the melancholic quest which was characterized by fleeting joy followed by the pang of separation from the object of the quest. These are things I gleaned from reading Corbin Scott Carnell's book *Bright Shadow of Reality: C. S. Lewis and the Feeling Intellect*. I remember being highly suspicious that Carnell's ponderous book was really a doctoral thesis in disguise. Now that I am able to search for it online, I find my suspicion to be substantiated.

Lab Experiment #11, April 24, 1980
Vertebrate Physiology

Notes: The human heart. Electrocardiology (EKG) is rather involved. Electrical axis of the heart spreads from negative to positive. Lead #1 on left arm and right arm. Lead #2 on right arm and left leg. Lead #3 on left leg and left arm. These three leads converge around the triangle of vectors, or Ivonger's Triangle, of the heart. The direction charge is running over the heart and is a sum of all three leads. There is a spreading of the depolarization wave, with the vector running down towards the left foot. The direction can change when something is wrong with the heart. For this lab, only turn in vector analysis.

Psychophysiology of Religion

William James contends that personal religious experience has its root and center in mystical states of consciousness, a shifting of the inner equilibrium, a breaking down of the walls of inhibition very similar to hypnotic states. In medical evaluations of mystical states, they appear to be imitated hypnotic states and a form of hysteria. James concludes this after conducting experiments—on himself—using nitrous oxide, or laughing gas.

C. S. Lewis

"If love is only lust, religion only aberrant psychology, thought only cerebral biochemistry, and the universe only a mathematical construct, the world would not be the rich and wild and startling place it manifestly is," writes Carnell in his English Literature dissertation-turned-book. At age nineteen, I do like this turn of phrase and feel he has made a valid point. I am not sure I want to proceed in life—whether or not as a scientist—without believing in something beyond what I can prove exists. But that increasingly does not equate with having any organized religion as part of my life. And especially not any religion headed by a male deity.

At the time, I did not make the connection between my wavering faith and my fraught relationship with my father. I do make that connection now.

Lab Experiment #12, May 8, 1980
Vertebrate Physiology

Notes: Schneider's Physical Fitness Test. Start with using phonocardiogram to record lab partner's heart sounds: *lub-dub. Lub* is the first sound and is due to more than one thing, but predominantly it is caused by the closing of the atrioventricular (AV) valves. *Dub* is the second sound and is mostly caused by closing of the aortic valves. Sounds between these two are termed murmurs. Take blood pressure and pulse rate at rest and then immediately after exercise (running up and down the stairs two times). Results: My resting blood pressure was 112/60 and my resting heart rate was 52. Immediately after exercise, my blood pressure was 135/70 and my heart rate was 128. Both blood pressure and heart rate returned to baseline after three minutes of rest.

Psychophysiology of Religion

Darwin's theory of evolution fit right in with the religion of nature and with the waning Romanticism. As an optimistic theology, meliorism can be summed up with the sunny survival-of-the-fittest statement: God is well, and so are you. This fed into the Progressive Era, but meliorism was dealt a fatal blow by the rise of Nazism, World War II, and the evidence of Nazi atrocities presented during the Nuremburg trials.

C. S. Lewis

Lewis believed that those persons who have bouts of melancholy have been cursed with a deformity which hampers biological fulfillment. Lewis included in *The Four Loves* the fact (according to him) that women spoil men's groups and therefore they should be kept separate. In my notes, I include multiple exclamation points beside this quotation. As I remember, it was at this point, on this exact day, when I decided that I was done reading C. S. Lewis.

Standing now, and again, at the intersection of objective science and subjective religion, I consult my version of a dashboard compass for navigation in life. My compass bears little resemblance to that of my Oberlin advisor and mentor, Professor Walker. My compass is composed of an amalgam of the questions and limits of both science and religion—questions and limits I continue to explore through my personal life and through my work as a nurse and feminist scholar. My compass is more like a crystal ball—or perhaps a snow globe containing Jadis, her Deplorable Word, her Minotaur and hags, and the entire *Oxford English Dictionary*.

Fifteen

Medical Maze

Who's turned us around like this,
so that whatever we do, we always have
the look of someone going away?
—Rainer Maria Rilke

Wayfinding

I work in the world's largest university building: the Warren G. Magnuson Health Sciences Building at the University of Washington (UW) in Seattle. The building, which includes the 450-bed UW Medical Center hospital, has close to six million square feet of space, the equivalent of more than thirty Walmart Supercenters, under one roof. The building comprises more than twenty wings, whose hallways are connected, but in a disorienting, Escherian way. Besides the hospital and its associated specialty clinics and administrative offices, the medical complex is home to five health science schools—medicine, nursing, dentistry, pharmacy, and public health. Ten thousand people work or are hospital patients in this building; many spend at least some time lost in the medical maze.

The UW medical complex is sandwiched between two busy streets and one busy ship canal. The building's courtyards are covered in concrete, with a few scraggly rhododendrons in containers. There are numerous entrances and exits to the building. Inside, the hallways have exposed guts—tangles of wires and pipes—and are lined with metal carts filled with glass test tubes, flasks, boxes of fruit flies, and cages of rats. The air is uniformly cold, with an acrid-medicinal, disinfectant smell. The bathrooms are tiled—floors and walls all the way to the ceiling—and the tiles are painted a jaundiced yellow. Some of the oldest rooms retain remnants of the original pale "hospital green" so popular in the twentieth century.

"Spinach green" is what Harry Sherman, a surgeon in a San Francisco hospital in 1914, named his invention. Using color theory, he distilled this green to counterbalance the hemoglobin red he encountered in his operating room. He claimed that this particular tone of green helped him discern anatomical details, resulting in better surgical outcomes. At around the same time, a leading American hospital architect, William O. Ludlow, advocated the use of color therapy: "The convalescent needs the positive colors that nature has spread so lavishly for her children . . . soft greens, pale blues . . . but above all, the glorious golden yellow of the sunshine." Perhaps the pale-yellow tiles and paint in the UW medical complex bathrooms started off the shade of sunshine, but they have not aged well.

Color-coding of medical center hallways and units helps people navigate the complex physical structure of the modern hospital and clinic. It is a form of wayfinding, which is a dynamic relationship to space, a continuous problem-solving process: knowing where you are and where you are headed, knowing and following the best route to get from here to there, and knowing when you have arrived at your destination. Large hospitals create a modern urban common space like no other. The closest parallels are probably busy airport terminals. But in hospitals, the business is not simply travel; the business of hospitals is life, illness, and death. Susan Sontag points out that we all hold dual citizenship, "in the kingdom of the well and in the kingdom of the sick." In hospitals, she states, patients are "emigrating to the kingdom of the ill."

The first time I entered the UW medical complex was in February 1994. I was visiting Seattle from Baltimore, where I was finishing my doctorate in global health. As a single mother of a seven-year-old son, I needed a stable, well-paying job—something global health did not offer. On a whim, I contacted the UW School of Nursing about a tenure-track academic position they had advertised. Teaching nursing was far down my list of desirable careers. I had long viewed nursing as old, stale, and a hindrance to my ambitions—yet when I am feeling more humble, I can't imagine a higher calling than being a nurse. I was, and still am, a nurse. Despite what I term my nursing ambivalence, I was curious about this job possibility. It helped that Seattle was as exotic as a foreign country to me.

"There's a courtyard on your right. You'll see a sculpture of people hanging on the outside wall of a brick building—go past that and enter the doors to your right."

These were the directions given to me by the professor with whom I'd set up an informational interview. I found her office, had a series of interviews, was offered and accepted the job. So, in December of that same year, after moving across the country to start my new job and new life in a new city, I went to my first official day of work. I parked in the cavernous underground S1 parking lot behind the medical complex. I followed the cute little tooth signs out of the parking lot, through a tunnel, and into the dental school entrance. Knowing the general direction I needed to go to get to my new office, I took the stairs up one floor and then decided to take a shortcut through a small internal courtyard. I suddenly found myself locked inside a ten-by-ten-foot barren cement courtyard that was surrounded on all sides by six stories of brick walls. I stood there for several minutes, gazing up at the walls, contemplating escape scenarios, contemplating the possible deeper meaning of this space, awed by its quiet peacefulness, before a woman passed by and opened the door for me. I have never been able to find that courtyard again—it doesn't exist on any map.

Today, I am a tenured associate professor in the Department of Psychosocial and Community Health in the UW School of Nursing. No one knows what the word *psychosocial* really means, including me, so I tell people I work in the Department of Community Health. As of December 2014, I have officially worked here for twenty years.

My office is in the ugliest wing of the medical complex. The wing's hallways are painted the same sick yellow as the bathrooms. There is a six-inch-wide gray rubber seam that bisects my office. It runs up one wall, across the ceiling, down the other wall, and across the floor. This rubber seam is the building's earthquake shock absorber. I often wonder what it would be like to stand on the rubber fault line during an earthquake. Would I be safer there rather than under my fake-wood desk or trying to find my way out of the building?

The particular part of the Health Sciences Building I work in, the T-Wing, was built in the late 1960s and is a prime example of brutalism. It is also a prime example of why brutalism is not an architectural style suited either for Seattle weather or for being attached to a hospital. Brutalism was an architectural movement that espoused the use of exposed concrete and other functional elements. It focused on the ideals of a better future through the use of technology.

Outside and inside the T-Wing, the building appears to be made of crumbling, damp, and moldy concrete. In one staircase I use frequently, there are arm-sized stalactites on the ceiling, with liquid perpetually oozing from their pointed ends down into a black and green puddle on a stair landing. It has a bizarre beauty. Every few years, someone from the maintenance crew removes the stalactites and paints the ceiling. I watch as the stalactites slowly return.

The land that the UW medical complex is built on had been salmon fishing ground for the Lakes Duwamish people before white settlers claimed it as pastureland for cows. As the town of Seattle grew, and the UW moved from its original downtown location north to its current location, the forty-acre parcel of land became a nine-hole golf course, then the 1909 Alaska-Yukon-Pacific Exposition's Pay Streak section with carnival rides, then briefly the site of a World War I navy training camp, and finally it became the site of the expanding Health Sciences and University Hospital. On October 9, 1949, Governor Arthur B. Langlie laid a ceremonial cornerstone for the official opening of the Health Sciences Building. Inside the cornerstone was a lead box containing a stethoscope, a set of false teeth, a nurse's cap, and a mortar and pestle: artifacts representing the Schools of Medicine, Dentistry, Nursing, and Pharmacy, which were housed in the new building. The box with the artifacts is still there.

Cornerstone, foundation stone, quoin stone: the first stone set for a new building. The stone that all others are set in reference to. The stone that determines the strength and future stability of the building. The stone that holds the genius loci, the guardian spirit, of the place.

Threshold

The modern hospital traces its roots back to Greek temples of healing, which were often caves set near streams or pools of water. There was an elaborate set of initiations that ill people went through in order to enter the sacred space of healing from the outside profane world. Bathing and the donning of clean, flowing robes. Going barefoot and ridding oneself of rings or other jewelry. Then being given a pallet in a large, communal sleeping place, an *enkoimeteria*, where patients slept side by side as they were to do centuries later in open hospital wards.

The Greek temples of healing had stone tablets, *iamata*, set outside the entrances. The tablets were inscribed with healing narratives—testimonials—in the form of poetry or brief prose, all written in third person. Ancient Greek healing practices included bathing, exercise, special diets, dream divination, and bloodletting. Prayers at an altar at the threshold, the entrance to the healing space. Sacrifices of animals and offerings of food.

The business of hospitals, in ancient Greece as well as now, is life, illness, and death. Everyone who enters the hospital as a patient emigrates—at least temporarily—to the land of the sick. It is a shadowland, a liminal space where tides ebb and flow, a place that offers glimpses of the abyss. As the surgeon Richard Selzer points out, a hospital is alive: "The walls palpitate to the rhythm of its heart, while in and out the window fly daydreams and nightmares. It is a dynamism that is transmitted to the hospital by the despair and the yearning of the sick."

Arrival

Late one November night in 2000, I drove myself to the emergency room at the UW Medical Center. I had left my twelve-year-old son sleeping at home. Still a single mother, I had called my boyfriend to come over and stay while I was gone.

My legs had been tingling and getting progressively benumbed over the past week. The numbness started in my toes and now reached my butt and groin region, plus my toes were turning blue. I had no idea what was wrong. The weekend before, I had run up the two thousand four hundred feet to the top of Mount Constitution on Orcas Island in the Puget Sound. It had been cold on the mountain, but I hadn't fallen or gotten frostbite. I was forty and in decent shape, was rarely ever sick, and had no primary care doctor. I worked as a nurse practitioner at a nearby community health clinic; I was used to diagnosing and treating other people's health problems, not my own.

"Take off all your clothes except your underwear and put them in this bag. And tie the gown in the back," the ER nurse said, as she handed me a cotton gown and a white plastic bag marked "University of Washington Medical Center: Patient Belongings" in purple. *Why did I wear black thong underwear to the ER?* I thought, as I gazed down at my mottled blue toes.

My personal mantra at the time was "I can do this; I can do anything!" I didn't see the danger in that saying. I worked three jobs, trying to pay off school debts and save for a down payment on a house, as well as for my son's future college education. I had been running on the tenure track, applying for and getting research grant after research grant, publishing a string of papers, collecting teaching and peer evaluations. The faculty had recently met to decide whether or not to grant me tenure. I didn't yet know the outcome. If I did not get tenure, I would lose my main job. So, there in the ER I did as I was told, stripped to my underwear, donned the gown smelling strongly of bleach, and then endured a series of tests and examinations. At some point, although I don't remember when, a plastic hospital ID band was strapped to my left wrist over the spot where my silver bracelets had been.

Covered by a white sheet up to my chin, I was now lying flat on my back on a black-plastic-encased gurney, *perhaps one that has recently delivered a dead body downstairs to the morgue. Can I feel my legs? Are they still there or have they been amputated? Or is it just that they are frozen, because I'm so cold? What time is it and why are we going through all these hallways?*

The air around me was cold—refrigerated-morgue cold—and filled with the low murmuring of disembodied voices, accompanied by the white noise whooshing of the building's ventilation system. Overhead, flashing, blindingly bright rectangles of fluorescent ceiling lights marched along in single file. I began counting them, memorizing the pathway so I could find my way back out again. Lines of closed doors whirred past on either side. No windows. No wall clocks. *I can't feel my legs. What time is it?* I tried to lift my head up off the thin pillow to look at my legs, to look for a clock, but I was too tired. *Have they given me medication to knock me out?*

A burly male orderly was behind my head, pushing my body on the gurney through the hallways. I could see long nose hairs in his cavernous nostrils and smell occasional wafts of stale coffee breath. He didn't speak. As we passed people in the hallways, white-coated and blue-scrub-wearing staff members, they all stopped briefly, turned sideways, backs against the walls, to let us pass. They furtively glanced down at my face, but their eyes always flitted away, never making eye contact.

I thought of Kafka's *Metamorphosis* as I lay flat on that hospital gurney being wheeled through numerous hallways, then wheeled into an extra-wide elevator lined with rubber bumpers, and then upstairs to the neurology floor of the hospital and checked in by a sweet young nurse who greeted me as Dr. Ensign and I realized she had been one of my students in a health systems course taught the previous spring in a large auditorium I think I was rolled past on this gurney on my way up here—*but that can't be right*. I had started thinking in run-on sentences. This young nurse, my student, handed me a tiny plastic cup filled with lilac-colored liquid. I looked at her, trying to remember if she was the sort of student I could trust to give me the right medication. Then I swallowed the saccharine-sweet syrup with a metallic aftertaste. I awoke in a darkened room with a spotlight directed at my right arm, some young man thumping my veins and then drawing tube after tube of dark-red blood.

After three days of hospital MRIs, X-rays, spinal taps, more blood draws, nerve-conduction tests on my legs, and totally annoying flashing light tests in my eyes, the gray-bearded senior attending neurologist appeared in my hospital room, accompanied by a fluttering group of neophyte short-white-coated medical students. He told me that the good news was that they had ruled out a spinal tumor, but the bad news was that I had autoimmune transverse myelitis, meaning my body was allergic to itself and was causing a swelling of my lower spine.

"We'll have to wait and see what it develops into. It can take a year or so before it progresses enough to make a definitive diagnosis," the neurologist said, peering at me over his rectangular wire-framed glasses.

So, I went home and waited. I desperately wanted a diagnosis, a unifying name for the bizarre collection of symptoms that kept sneaking up and sprouting into new signs—the concrete objective markers—and symptoms—the soft subjective *could be all in my head; could be just female hysteria*. Symptoms such as my favorite: malaise, a general feeling of being unwell. *Malaise*, from the Old French *mal* ("bad") and *aise* ("ease"), space, elbow room. I was in a bad space. I had not understood what it felt like to be in a body that betrayed me. I thought a diagnosis could bring me back into my body, bring me back into a good space.

The numbness slowly resolved, although my toes continued to turn blue, as did my fingers. Then all my joints began to swell. I spent the next year going to various specialists and subspecialists, one of whom drew fourteen tubes of blood all in one visit, to run a panel of obscure and insanely expensive tests, from which the results were inconclusive. Another specialist drew my blood, extracted the serum, and injected it into my forearm to measure my body's allergic reaction—to myself.

I tried complementary medicine and went to an acupuncturist who had been an internal medicine physician but had burned out on working within the medical system. He told me the story of his final days in medicine: "I told the administration that I wouldn't take it anymore and I walked out," he said. "Now don't move because I'm going very close to your heart," he added as he jammed a large needle into the middle of my sternum. A large purple bruise bloomed on my chest for weeks afterwards, taking my mind off my blue toes and swollen joints.

I was grateful for my university-sponsored health insurance, but was tired of all the medical encounters that seemed only to lead to more medical encounters. What I dubbed my "mystery illness" morphed into a diagnosis of mixed connective tissue disease (MCTD), which is really something that can't make up its mind between being lupus, or rheumatoid arthritis, or the totally freaky-scary scleroderma, where your skin and internal organs thicken and petrify while you are still alive. MCTD is a rare autoimmune disorder that attacks the fibers providing the framework and support for the body. *Rare, as in I'm special? Or as in I'm cursed?* I thought, as a specialist explained my diagnosis, my dis-ease, my mal-aise. As he told me my diagnosis, my world closed in, like the bedroom doors closing on Kafka's man-turned-beetle.

Today, my medical chart still lists a diagnosis of MCTD, but none of the freaky-scary petrifying stuff has occurred. I no longer run the medical circuit in search of more tests, more tubes of blood, more diagnoses, more jabs to the heart, more promises of a cure. I live with it as you would live with a curmudgeonly, truth-telling friend. It tells me when I'm falling back into the inhuman *I can do it; I can do anything!* mindset. I listen to my body, even as it continues to get lost in the impossible hallways at work.

Most of the time, I embrace the stalactites, the career limbo of nursing ambivalence, and the bewildering staircases. Recently, I cleaned out my university office and recycled all my papers, academic books, and grant reports. I prepared to slow down my tenure-track conveyor belt, step into a sabbatical, search for that tranquil courtyard that doesn't exist on any map.

I chose a soft, calming color for the walls of my office. Then, after the maintenance crew had repainted the walls, I realized I had picked a version of hospital green. I've decided to live with it, and to see what fine details of life it reveals.

Sixteen

Degree of Latitude

There is wild in us yet, and in every word and sentence and speech there is still the seethe of the sea from which we came, and from which we will return.
—Brian Doyle

This is a test of your mental state.

1. Where are you right now? (But first: Who are you? What's the story of your true name?)
2. What's the date—day, month, year? (Where did you come from and where are you headed?)
3. Repeat these three words after me: whale, map, stone. (Don't question them; they're important words.)
4. Spell world backwards. (Now spell world spinning.)
5. Repeat the phrase: "A rolling stone gathers no moss." What do you suppose it means? (Be careful of your answer. It can indicate instability.)
6. Take these stones in your right hand. Roll them slowly in your hand like dice. Drop them on the floor. (Repeat. Gently, rhythmically. Imagine ocean waves lapping the shores of a pebbled beach.)
7. Write a sentence. (Now write another sentence connected with the first. Repeat.)
8. Tell me the names of the three items I gave you earlier. (Remember them? Whale, map, stone . . .)

Whale

August 11, 1980. Time: 17:20 / Position: 49.39 degrees N, 60.29 degrees W. Sea level. Banc Beaugé, Gulf of Saint Lawrence, Canada.

Call me Josephine, although at the time I went by my childhood nickname: BJ. I've just turned nineteen and am at the helm of the *Westward*, a 125-foot topsail schooner oceanographic research vessel out of Woods Hole, Cape Cod, Massachusetts. We're under full sail. I'm steering a course southeast towards Lark Harbour, Bay of Islands, Newfoundland. I glance down at the glass-globe crystal ball of the compass binnacle in front of me. We've been blown off course by a force 9 gale lasting two days and nights. Today it's passed by to the north, leaving us in sight of the desolate, flat-lined coast of Labrador. The heavy gray clouds undulate above us, breaking in places to lapis sky. The breeze is stiff and steady, whipping small white-frothed waves against our hull.

The air smells of briny salt, earthy teak from the ship's decking, and tobacco. Standing beside me is Captain Chase, whose chiseled profile, neatly trimmed blond mustache, and pipe are in my peripheral vision. He's gazing ahead when a low siren explosion sounds to our port side, accompanied by a thirty-foot-tall spout of seawater. The breeze changes to include a fetid fish smell. There's a seventy-foot blue whale just yards from our boat. The captain calmly yells a command to prepare to come about.

We're part of an ongoing study of whales in the Gulf of Saint Lawrence and have seen numerous pods of pilot whales along with minke, fin, and humpback whales. But this is our first sighting of a blue whale, *Balaenoptera musculus*. They're elusive, solitary, and migratory. They're also the largest animals ever to have lived on earth—almost twice as large as the largest land or sea dinosaur. No photograph, no video—not even 3-D IMAX—can come close to replicating the feeling of being there. It's awesome; it's awful.

This isn't my big fish tale. What's important is the context, the exact location, the time, the sea, and landmarks, of a fixed point of memory I've carried with me. Why do some memories stay and others flee?

Map

In the early 1990s I worked with teens who were thrownaway, runaway, tossed about, and spat out onto the menacing streets of Baltimore. To the huddled small groups in emergency shelters I gave colored markers, stickers, and large sheets of paper, and I asked them to draw a map of their neighborhood—wherever it was in Baltimore that they were most familiar. Their maps always included Charles Street as their north-south meridian. They were either East or West Baltimoreans. For many of the teens, their parents and grandparents had never ventured across Charles Street, had never traveled outside their immediate neighborhoods. They didn't find this strange.

I was a nurse working on my doctorate in international public health. I'd wanted to become a biologist, a naturalist who studied the migratory patterns of fish and whales; instead, I'd become a nurse. I'd been thrown off course. But now I was finding my way back.

We develop cognitive maps—mental maps, mind's-eye maps—through exploring our environment, studying actual maps, and hearing information about our world. The community mapping I did with Baltimore teens charted their mental maps. I asked them to locate their main hangout areas, to tell me why some were safe and others unsafe. At the time, Baltimore had the highest murder rate of any city in the United States, one of the highest rates in the world. For these young people, their maps were urban warfare tactical maps—strategies for survival.

I rowed a single in the waters of Baltimore. Balanced in a sleek racing shell, holding a sculling oar in each hand, I navigated around orange-buoyed Superfund contamination sites, submerged ships and refrigerators, and through curtains of dangling chicken necks suspended by crab-hunting strings beneath low-lying bridges. The air I breathed while rowing smelled of urine, iron, and rotten flesh. On our rowing house dock, my feet crunched waves of tiny glass crack vials washed up by the tide. I memorized the maps of the Patapsco River, and of the Middle Branch and Inner Harbor waters I rowed. I can still tell you exactly where the shoal of dumped appliances lies.

Buried deep inside our brains, in the primitive limbic system, are cells that record our movement, our navigation through time and space: place cells, grid cells, border cells. These are our mental map cells. The way the brain records and remembers movement in space appears to be the basis of all memory. Place cells encode spatial information layered with sensory input from our environment to become associated with particular experiences: memories. We are born with rudimentary internal cognitive maps that we add to over our lifetimes, creating a mosaic of map-bits and scene constructions.

The memory of the briefest of events can last a lifetime. Where on the coordinates of our memory maps do our first memories reside? Do these first memories define us? Do they point us in specific directions? In mine I am three. It's late afternoon of a rainy summer day in Virginia. I'm lying in bed, swaddled in the primordial smell of moist humus and the lush leafy gleam coming from the open windows. On the green shag rug are pieces of white typing paper with penciled scribbles. I'm alone in my room, drowsy, deeply, achingly content.

Stone

They are my runes, my lots. The memory, the fixed point, is embedded in two white stones I've carried with me since finding them in the waters of the blue whale. These are my Jonah's stones. They didn't come from the whale; they came from the inner ears of a large white cod caught in nets while we sampled the pink krill the whale was feeding on. I was studying the swim bladders—primitive lungs—and inner ears of bony fish.

The stones are called *otoliths*: Greek for "ear stones." All vertebrates, including humans, have otoliths, although some, like ours, are microscopic. The stones are suspended in fluid in the labyrinths of the inner ear. They aid in perception of sound and gravitational forces, in maintenance of balance and orientation—of direction. Otoliths are part of ultrasonic speech perception in humans: we can discern speech beyond our hearing range. Listen carefully to that fact. Do you hear voices others can't hear?

We are more influenced by our physical environment than we are comfortable acknowledging. Sensory stimuli that we filter out or that are present below a detectable level influence our decisions, induce subliminal learning, and are stored with specific memories. Place is part of us; place lives in us.

My otoliths, the two from the white cod, live in a small tin pillbox, with the image of an English thatched-roof cottage printed on it. I bought the tin in a small fishing village built on stilts along the pebbled edge of a tranquil Newfoundland fjord. The otoliths are pearly white, curled like mummified embryos. Similar to seashells, they're composed of calcium carbonate absorbed from the waters, their layers analogous to growth rings of trees: a new layer for each year of life. The otoliths have stayed with me, have become my talismans.

Take these stones in your right hand. Roll them slowly in your hand like dice. Drop them on the floor. (Repeat. Gently, rhythmically. Imagine ocean waves lapping the shores of a pebbled beach.)
Remember them? Whale, map, stone . . .

March 27, 2014. Time: 13:30 / Position: 35.58 degrees S, 173.30 degrees E. Sea level. Waimamaku Beach, Northland, New Zealand.

Call me Josephine. This is the story of my true name.

I'm fifty-three years old and am floating naked in a rock pool filled with cold water from the Tasman Sea. The low tide has exposed large slabs of black volcanic rock—basalt scoria with frozen-in-time bubbles of Miocene-era lava gas. The rocks shelter me from the open sea. Fine salt mist from the crashing waves settles on my face, my lips, my tongue. Above me are layers of leaden gray clouds. In the rock pool are small bright purple and orange crabs, silver minnows, pink sea fans, green-lipped mussels, and burnt-orange starfish. On the exposed rocks above me are fringes of chartreuse-green sea lettuce, undulating dreadlocks of dun-green sea kelp, and a flock of orange-beaked, pink-footed oystercatchers. I'm cradled in an impossibly psychedelic crayon-colored landscape. I arch my back, duck my head below water, and emerge to see that it is real; I am not drunk or on drugs or crazy.

Spell world *backwards. (Now spell world spinning.)*

The night before, I stood on a treeless hilltop studying the clear nighttime sky. Far from any city lights, the sky was ink black, startling in proximity of stars and Milky Way. As I searched for Orion, the anchor for me in direction-finding at night, I realized the constellation was upside down, rotated and reversed left to right. It lies in the northern sky, versus the southern for me at home in the Northern Hemisphere. And, forgetting where I was, I looked in vain for the Big Dipper and the North Star, before recognizing the Southern Cross. Inside the Milky Way were small white puffs I first mistook for passing clouds, and then realized were galaxies I'd never seen.

Entering a new and dramatic territory can make us realize the potency of place; it can make us sense our embodiment of place. While being within such a dislocating experience, we are literally and figuratively out of place. That's what happened to me on the hilltop that night. I stood outside for hours trying to regain my bearings, my balance, my location. Only the growing awareness of being stung by silent stealth mosquitoes brought me back to my body, to the ground beneath my bare feet, and to my bed with dreams of new geographies.

Repeat the phrase: "A rolling stone gathers no moss." What do you suppose it means? (Be careful of your answer. It can indicate instability.)

A common brain network underlies memory and imagination, including future thinking. Both are mental time travel. Past events of great importance that shape a person's sense of identity are manifested similarly in the construction of self-defining future projects and experiences; they are self-defining and directional memories. Since the past and the future are part of us, it is not only the present that matters.

I'm at the end of my three-month stay in New Zealand. I've just finished teaching a university study-abroad program with sixteen college juniors—all young women. They returned home to Seattle last week, taking with them their questions about careers and future trajectories. Floating in the rock pool beside the Tasman Sea, I ask myself a question I posed to my students at the end of their journeys: *Where did you come from and where are you headed?*

In the still point between the crashing waves of the wild Tasman Sea, I know that this is my self-defining, directional memory as it is being made: a memory I know I will have even while it is—and was—occurring.

Write a sentence. (Now, write another sentence connected with the first. Repeat.)

Epilogue

As I write this, in mid-June of 2017, at the end of my first postsabbatical academic year, I continue to search for that tranquil courtyard in my own life and work—the courtyard I became locked inside when I was first learning to navigate my way through the university health sciences complex where I work. In my recent annual review meeting with my department chair, I asked for ideas of good places to write within the sprawling health sciences complex. I was hoping for a quiet and hidden storage room sufficiently far enough away from the formaldehyde-emanating human-cadaver dissection rooms on the floors above my office. She thought for a moment and then replied, "Your office here in our department. When it was my office, that's where I could write NIH grant applications and reports. Or perhaps a study carrel in the Health Sciences Library."

After the meeting, I decided to try to write in the Health Sciences Library in the basement below my office. I had already tried many times to write in my university office—my office with the hospital spinach-green walls—and it had not worked out well. Its *genius loci* ghost was not conducive to creative pursuits, to real writing. So, I found myself sitting in a worn-out wooden desk carrel in a windowless back corner of the library, in amongst floor-to-ceiling metal shelves filled with medical reference books. It was during the late-spring university break, so I was alone in the room.

I went to the library that day not only to write, but also to return an ancient, crumbling copy of William James's *The Varieties of Religious Experience*—a book I had checked out and reread in order to research and write my essay on science and religion, "Lab Notebook," now included in *Soul Stories*. I held on to James's book much longer than was necessary, to have it serve as a sort of humanistic talisman in my office at work.

Surrounding me in the library were books on sleep disorders (amusingly juxtaposed with large No Sleeping Allowed Here! signs on the walls), next to books on memory disorders and anxiety disorders (*Why Zebras Don't Get*

Ulcers was part of a catchy title), and one lone book on resilience that perhaps was misshelved. And, in a bookcase nearby, there was an entire section of family therapy books. *Perhaps I have found my proper niche here*, I thought. *But where are the real books? Where are the patient illness stories, the philosophy, art, history, and health humanities books? And where am I located within this space?* I asked myself.

Personality disorders had its own section near family therapy. I noticed one textbook, titled *Broken Structures*, that was about severe personality disorders. *There but by the grace of god, time, therapy—and reflective writing—go I*, I thought. I realized that I was searching in this physical space not only for a place to write, but also for ways to incorporate the stories of health and healing (including my own illness stories) into health care and into health provider education. Where in this medical maze of the Health Sciences Library were there examples of these?

As I wandered through the shelves filled with bound medical journals and books, I stumbled upon a small section of books in a dark corner near the cobwebbed rear emergency exit. This section included Susan Sontag's book *Illness as Metaphor*, medical artwork books, books on the mental illnesses of famous writers (including, curiously enough, Florence Nightingale), and multiple biographies and memoirs about and by physicians. Also, there was a fascinating book on the medieval artistic genre the dance of death, with many pieces of artwork to illustrate the changes throughout history of the "danse macabre" (as it is known in French). There were intriguing examples of artwork illustrating the dance of death as applied to the modern plague of HIV/AIDS. The purpose of the danse macabre is to serve as a reminder of the fact that all of us—no matter our station in life—will ultimately face illness and death.

Upstairs, on my way out of the library, tucked in a corner in the reserves section, next to the bone boxes and hanging human skeletons (forming their own danse macabre still life), were two well-thumbed copies of my medical memoir, *Catching Homelessness*. My book was experiencing its last few days as the UW Health Sciences Common Book. The Common Book is part of our health humanities program across the six health science schools. I had located at least a part of myself, tattered and dog-eared and coffee-stained though it was.

My search for that tranquil courtyard that doesn't exist on any map continues and perhaps intensifies. During my review meeting with my department chair, I had the fleeting vision of setting up a table in a hallway of the Health Sciences Building and writing there, perhaps invoking a version of the *Get Smart* Cone of Silence: nurse writer as performance art. I am still searching for ways to incorporate—and to sustain—the arts and humanities in my professional life. For now, it appears that the main place to nurture those is here: at home, in my own office, overlooking my bamboo-shaded courtyard.

Ironically though, I now find myself writing another grant proposal—not to the National Institutes of Health for research, but rather a proposal for population health funding to develop, implement, and evaluate a community café in the University District where our Seattle campus is located. Modeled after the Merge Café in Auckland, New Zealand, this community café would address food and housing insecurity, as well as mental and physical health and well-being. It would be designed to provide a safe space for being unsafe, for community members—housed and unhoused—university health science and other students, and staff and faculty members to sit down together at a large community table, share food and stories and creative writing and artwork. And to build a capacity for empathy, for true resilience, for endurance, and for work towards health equity and social justice.

I am reminded of physician and narrative medicine scholar Sayantani DasGupta's wise words in her essay "Narrative Medicine, Narrative Humility: Listening to the Streams of Stories." In her essay, DasGupta describes her work in narrative medicine as teaching people to listen:

> What I'm ultimately interested in is teaching people to listen critically, to listen in socially just ways. I want to teach health care providers to listen not only to comfortable stories, or stories of folks who are just like them, but also stories that challenge them, stories that are from the margins, stories that are traditionally silenced.

My hope is that the essays, poems, and resources included in *Soul Stories: Voices from the Margins* help move us in that direction.

—Seattle, Washington

Acknowledgments

The experience of writing a book such as this is, as George Orwell so aptly described, quite a lot like having a long, serious illness or a bout of demon-possession. It requires the care and support of an entire village to live through—to endure. There is the work of writing a book, and then there is the added work of writing a book about trauma, including one's own childhood trauma. My village for this book included first and foremost my life partner, Peter Kahn, and my two amazingly wise young adult children, Jonathan Bowdler and Margaret Kahn.

I also want to acknowledge the generous support of the University of Washington Simpson Center for the Humanities and the National Endowment for the Humanities—without their support, this book and the accompanying digital *Soul Stories* transmedia project would not be possible. Thank you to the anonymous reviewers at the National Endowment for the Humanities Public Scholars Program for their reflective critiques of early drafts of parts of the *Soul Stories* manuscript. My colleague, medical anthropologist Lorna Rhodes, provided me with welcome feedback and suggestions as I wrote the essay "Endurance Test" included in this book.

Thanks to the amazing librarians at the University of Washington, especially Joanne Rich in the Health Sciences Library, for helping me track down some of the more difficult-to-find sources of information included in this book, and Anne Davis in the Odegaard Library, for her assistance with my *Soul Stories* multimedia installation during winter and spring quarters of 2015.

Additional support for my *Soul Stories* project came from 4Culture and the Jack Straw Productions' 2013 Jack Straw Writers Program, curated by the talented and generous Stephanie Kallos. It was during this program that the idea for *Soul Stories* came into existence, and it was through my interactions with the creative group of Jack Straw writers that my writing was deepened and enriched. My gratitude also extends to Hedgebrook for giving me the "radical hospitality" of a writers-in-residence retreat in the fall of 2014. Being in the company of a group of gifted, diverse, and radical women provided the support necessary for me to tell my story and to tell it in the way it needed to be told.

Portions of this book have appeared in print in different forms:

An earlier version of "Soul Story" was published in *The Jack Straw Writers Anthology* 17 (May 2013): 23–27.

"Witness: On Telling" was published in *Intima: A Journal of Narrative Medicine*, Fall 2017, available at http://www.theintima.org/field-notes-mz/.

"Listen, Carefully" was published as a 55-word story in "The Diagnosis Issue," ed. Annemarie Jutel, special issue, *Perspectives in Biology and Medicine* 58, no. 1 (Winter 2015): 32. It was published in its full-length version in Electric Literature's *Okey-Panky*, November 7, 2016, https://electriclitera-ture.com/listen-carefully-ea15e3a8e13e.

"Steps to Foot Care" was published in *Intima: A Journal of Narrative Medicine*, Spring 2014, available at http://www.theintima.org/fiction-mz/.

"Way Out; Way Home" was published in *Raven Chronicles Journal* 23 (2016): 160–67.

"Medical Maze" was published in *Intima: A Journal of Narrative Medicine*, Spring 2016, available at http://www.theintima.org/nonfiction-mz/.

"Degree of Latitude" was published by *Manifest-Station: On Being Human*, February 5, 2017, http://www.themanifeststation.net/?s=ensign.

Narrative Medicine Resources

The following are my favorite resources related to narrative medicine and the health humanities:

- NYU School of Medicine's medical humanities website (http://medhum.med.nyu.edu/) has a searchable database to reviews and sources of published works of literature, art, movies. They also maintain an email list and a blog.
- The International Health Humanities Network "bringing the human back into health" (at http://www.healthhumanities.org/). They describe their work this way:

The International Health Humanities Network provides a global platform for innovative humanities scholars, medical, health and social care professionals, voluntary sector workers and creative practitioners to join forces with informal and family carers, service-users and the wider self-caring public to explore, celebrate and develop new approaches in advancing health and well-being through the arts and humanities in hospitals, residential and community settings.

- The Brits have a much better health care system than we do, and they have a creative collection (is it a book? is it a collage?) on medical humanities. Published by the Wellcome Collection, *Where Does It Hurt? The New World of the Medical Humanities* is both entertaining and thought-provoking. (Available at: https://wellcomecollection.org/wheredoesithurt.) While you're at it, spend some time browsing their website for fun quizzes, interactive educational games, videos, and more. Here is what they say about the book:

What does it mean to be well? Or ill? And who, apart from you, really knows which is which? Contemporary definitions of medicine and clinical practice occupy just one small corner of a vast field of beliefs, superstitions, cultures and practices across which human beings have always roamed in the search to keep themselves, and others, feeling well. The label "medical humanities" is the best effort we've made so far to define the fence that encloses that very large field; recognising that it's a space in which artists, poets, historians, film-makers, comedians and cartoonists—in fact every one of us—has as much right to explore as any humanities-schooled or clinically trained professional. This book is a walk through that field, a celebration of its rich diversity, a dip into some of the conversations that are going on within it, an attempt to get it in perspective—and an invitation to you to join the conversation yourself.

- The health policy journal *Health Affairs* has a feature titled "Narrative Matters," which are personal essays written by patients, their families, and caregivers with a health policy aspect. *Health Affairs* has been running these essays for fifteen or so years, and they are a popular feature, crossing over to news features on *NPR* and in the *New York Times*. The editors of "Narrative Matters" published a book collection of forty-six of their best essays: Fitzhugh Mullan and Ellen Ficklen, editors, *Narrative Matters: The Power of the Personal Essay in Health Policy* (Baltimore: The Johns Hopkins University Press, 2006).
- *Bellevue Literary Review: A Journal of Humanity and Human Experience*. This is a print and online literary journal published by the Department of Medicine, NYU Langone Health. (Available at: http://blr.med.nyu.edu/.) They also have archived historical photos from Bellevue Hospital, the oldest continuously running hospital in the United States (although Hurricane Sandy in 2012 seriously affected their buildings and operation).
- *Creative Nonfiction*. This print journal is highly selective, only includes creative/narrative nonfiction, and is not primarily geared towards health-related writing. But the editor, Lee Gutkind, has focused much of his own writing on medical narratives.
- *Pulse: Voices from the Heart of Medicine* (https://pulsevoices.org/). As they state, *Pulse* is "an online magazine that uses stories and poems

from patients and health care professionals to talk honestly about giving and receiving medical care." You can sign up to get a weekly short essay or poem, as well as artwork and photographs. They have published print book anthologies, such as *Pulse: Voices from the Heart of Medicine, Editor's Picks—a Third Anthology*, edited by Paul Gross and Diane Guernsey (New Rochelle, NY: Voices from the Heart of Medicine, 2015).

- *The Examined Life Journal* from the University of Iowa Carver College of Medicine Writing and Humanities Program. This is a print journal; the college also holds an annual conference, The Examined Life Conference.

- *The Intima: A Journal of Narrative Medicine*, from the Columbia University Program in Narrative Medicine (http://www.theintima. org/). This is a beautifully done online narrative medicine journal.

- *Portfolio to Go: 1,000+ Reflective Writing Prompts and Provocations for Clinical Learners*, by Allan D. Peterkin (Toronto: University of Toronto Press, 2016). Besides containing a wide range of reflective writing prompts, Peterkin includes a chapter on "Guidelines for Narrative Accountability When Writing or Publishing About Patients/Clients" (chapter 34, pp. 154–56). This is an excellent guide to the murky ethical terrain involved in this sort of writing.

I include here a list of writing prompts that relate to the essays and poems included in Soul Stories. I arranged the prompts to follow the flow of the book, but some of the writing prompts do not necessarily belong to any one chapter.

1. Write about the last real thing that happened to you.
2. What draws you to the work that you do?
3. What are your biggest sources of potential (or real) professional burnout, and what can you do to either prevent, mitigate, or learn from them?
4. If your feet could talk, what would they say?
5. Pick two body parts (for instance, your eyes and your feet) and write an imaginary conversation that they might have with each other.
6. Write the story of your name. Now, write the story of your true

name. Do they differ? If so, how and why?

7. Write about something distasteful about a person (this can be a patient, a caregiver, a friend, a family member, or a public figure past or present) from a compassionate point of view.

8. Write of your first experience with death or loss of any kind.

9. Write the story of a scar you have. This can be a physical or emotional scar.

10. Think of the last time you perceived yourself as healthy. Describe the feeling and context using as much rich, descriptive detail as possible.

11. Write about the last time you felt deeply listened to.

12. Write about the first time you were aware of someone from another socioeconomic class than yours.

Notes

Epigraph

"**What kind of beast . . .**" Adrienne Rich, *The Dream of a Common Language* (New York: W. W. Norton, 1978), page 28.

Foreword

xi   "**Something else DasGupta writes**…" Sayantani DasGupta, "The Politics of Pedagogy: Cripping, Queering and Un-homing Health Humanities," in *The Principles and Practice of Narrative Medicine*, Rita Charon, Sayantani DasGupta, Nellie Hermann, Craig Irvine, Eric R. Marcus, Edgar Rivera Colón, Danielle Spencer, and Maura Spiegel (New York: Oxford University Press, 2017), 137-153.

Preface

xiii   "**Fortifies clinical practice with the narrative . . .**" Rita Charon, *Narrative Medicine: Honoring the Stories of Illness* (New York: Oxford University Press, 2006), page 4.

xiii–xiv **A narrative medicine close reading drill . . .** Charon, *Narrative Medicine*, 114–24.

xiv   "**Providing care that is respectful . . .**" Institute of Medicine (US) Committee on Quality of Health Care in America, *Crossing the Quality Chasm: A New Health System for the 21st Century, Executive Summary* (Washington, DC: National Academies Press, 2001), page 6.

xiv   **Charon concedes that the application . . .** Charon, *Narrative Medicine*, 67.

xiv   "**Choose the turning points . . .**" and "**Please share with me . . .**" Abigail Rasminsky, "The Doc Story: Her Philosophy Is Simple and Ancient, and It Could Change the Practice of Medicine," *O, The Oprah Magazine*,

July 2012, page 88.

xv   **"An archetypal story, which provides . . ."**   *Oxford English Dictionary*, s.v. "metanarrative," accessed May 1, 2017, http://www.oed.com.

xv   *Medical gaze* **is the term coined by . . .**   Michel Foucault, *The Birth of the Clinic: An Archaeology of Medical Perception* (New York: Vintage, 1993).

xv   **Irish physician Seamus O'Mahony calls "hinterland . . ."** Seamus O'Mahony, "Against Narrative Medicine," *Perspectives of Biology and Medicine* 56 (Autumn 2013): 611–19.

xvi   **"She calls for attention to…"**   Sayantani DasGupta, "The Politics of Pedagogy: Cripping, Queering and Un-homing Health Humanities," in *The Principles and Practice of Narrative Medicine*, Rita Charon, Sayantani DasGupta, Nellie Hermann, Craig Irvine, Eric R. Marcus, Edgar Rivera Colón, Danielle Spencer, and Maura Spiegel (New York: Oxford University Press, 2017), 137-138.

xvi   **"So when people say that poetry . . ."** Jeanette Winterson, *Why Be Happy When You Could Be Normal?* (New York: Grove Press, 2011), page 40.

xvii   **Similar to Roland Barthes's term** *punctum* **. . .**   Roland Barthes, *Camera Lucida: Reflections on Photography* (New York: Hill and Wang, 1981).

xvii   **As medical sociologist Arthur Frank states . . .** Arthur W. Frank, personal communication during the Narrative Research Methodology training workshop at the April 22, 2002, International Institute for Qualitative Methodology, Banff, Canada.

xviii   **I began to write what became . . .** Josephine Ensign, *Catching Homelessness: A Nurse's Story of Falling Through the Safety Net* (Berkeley: She Writes Press, 2016).

xix   **Health humanities is the relatively new field . . .** For more about health humanities, see The International Health Humanities Network http://www.healthhumanities.org/, the book by Paul Crawford, Brian Brown, Charley Baker, Victoria Tischler, and Brian Abrams, Health Humanities (New York: Palgrave Macmillan, 2015), as well as Paul Crawford, Brian Brown, Victoria Tischler, and Charley Baker, "Health Humanities: The Future of Medical Humanities?" *Mental Health Review Journal* 15, no. 3 (2010):4-10.

Soul Story

1   **"I love all waste . . ."** From the poem "Julian and Maddalo," by Percy
       Bysshe Shelley. In Percy Bysshe Shelley and H. Buxton Forman, eds., *The
       Works of Percy Bysshe Shelley in Verse and Prose: Now First Brought Together
       with Many Pieces Not Before Published* (London: Reeves and Turner,
       1880), pages 107-8.

1   **Leaning over a display case . . .** Mary Shelley, *The Journals of Mary
       Shelley*, eds. Paula R. Feldman and Diana Scott-Kilvert (Oxford:
       Clarendon Press, 1987).

2   **There was an exhibit,** *Shelley's Ghost* **. . .** The exhibit I saw in the New
       York Public Library was *Shelley's Ghost: Reshaping the Image of a Literary
       Family*, a collaborative exhibition by the Bodleian Libraries and the New
       York Public Library, http://shelleysghost.bodleian.ox.ac.uk/.

3   **The narrative medicine advanced workshop . . .** This workshop was
       offered by the Program in Narrative Medicine at the Columbia University
       College of Physicians and Surgeons, http://www.narrativemedicine.org/.

3   **Colm Toibin's short story . . .** Colm Toibin, "One Minus One," *The New
       Yorker*, May 7, 2007, http://www.newyorker.com/magazine/2007/05/07/
       one-minus-one.

5   **"Would rather wash the feet . . ." and "Makes for a bad nurse . . ."**
       Graham Greene, *A Burnt-Out Case* (New York: Penguin Books, 1975),
       page 22.

Walk in My Shoes

9   **"People often ask themselves the right questions . . ."** William
       Maxwell, *Time Will Darken It* (Boston: Nonpareil Books, 1948), page 86.

10   **"I could not give away . . ."** Joan Didion, *The Year of Magical Thinking*
       (New York: Vintage International, 2006), page 37.

12   **We tend to be more empathetic towards . . .** Lydia Lyle Gibson,
       "Mirrored Emotion," *The University of Chicago Magazine 98, no. 4*
       (April 2006), http://magazine.uchicago.edu/0604/features/emotion.
       shtml; Karsten Steuber, "Measuring Empathy," *Stanford Encyclopedia of
       Philosophy*, 2013, http://plato.stanford.edu/entries/empathy/measuring.
       html.

12   **I seldom am privy to . . .**   Daniel Chen, Robert Lew, Warren Hershman, and Jay Orlander, "A Cross-Sectional Measurement of Medical Student Empathy," *Journal of General and Internal Medicine 22* (February 19, 2007): 1434–38.

17   **"A penetration, a kind of travel . . ."** Leslie Jamison, *The Empathy Exams* (Minneapolis, MN: Graywolf Press), page 6.

18   **"Empathy can be a story you tell yourself . . ."** Rebecca Solnit, *The Faraway Nearby* (New York: Viking, 2013), page 106–7.

Witness: On Seeing

21   **"Bearing witness constitutes a specific form . . ."** Barbie Zelizer, *Remembering to Forget: Holocaust Memory Through the Camera's Eye* (Chicago: University of Chicago Press, 1998), page 10.

21   **"Witness a city in transformation . . ."** "52 Places to Go in 2014," *The New York Times*, January 1, 2014, http://www.nytimes.com/ interactive/2014/01/10/travel/2014-places-to-go.html.

22   **Over your cities grass will grow . . .** See Manohla Dargis's movie review of *Touring an Artist's Pre-Apocalyptic Realm: Over Your Cities Grass Will Grow*, directed by Sophie Fiennes, *The New York Times,* August 9, 2011, http://www.nytimes.com/2011/08/10/movies/over-your-cities-grass-will-grow-review.html.

23   **An art installation by Peter Majendie . . .** For a description of Peter Majendie's installation, see Elke Weesjes Sabella, "A Creative Rebirth: Public Art and Community Recovery in Christchurch," *Natural Hazards Observer* 40, no. 2 (November 28, 2015), https://hazards.colorado. edu/article/a-creative-rebirth-public-art-and-community-recovery-in-christchurch.

24   **Overwhelmed by the disaster tourism—thanatourism . . .** For a discussion of thanatourism, see Martin J. J. Murray, *Commemorating and Forgetting: Challenges for the New South Africa* (Minneapolis: University of Minnesota Press, 2013).

25   **"The feeling of being exempt from calamity . . ."** Susan Sontag, *On Photography* (New York: Farrar, Straus and Giroux, 1978), page 168.

25   **Inside is an interactive video installation . . .** Phil Dadson, *Bodytok Quintet: The Human Instrument Archive, Scape 7*, http://www. scapepublicart.org.nz/scape-7-bodytok-quintet/.

26   **"A word for the false sense of familiarity . . ."** Philip Armstrong, "On

Tenuous Grounds," *Landfall 222: Christchurch and Beyond* (November 2011): 8–19, page 8.

26   **Cameras are "clocks for seeing"** . . . Roland Barthes, *Camera Lucida: Reflections on Photography*, trans. Richard Howard (New York: Hill and Wang, a division of Farrar, Straus and Giroux, 2010), page 15.

26   **"While photographing subjects do not . . ."** "Code of Ethics," National Press Photographers Association, https://nppa.org/code_of_ethics.

27   **Kevin Carter, the white South African photographer . . .** For information on the photographer Kevin Carter, see Scott Macleod, "The Life and Death of Kevin Carter," *Time,* June 21, 2001, 70, http://content.time.com/time/magazine/article/0,9171,165071,00.html.

27   **The American photographer Diane Arbus . . .** For information on the photographer Diane Arbus, see Hal Hinson, "Arbus in Wonderland (Diane Arbus, Photographer)," *The Atlantic,* November 1984, 129; and Richard Woodward, "Shooting from the Hip," *ARTnews,* October 1, 2003, 106–9, http://www.artnews.com/2003/10/01/shooting-from-the-hip/.

28   **"I was an Ugly American Tourist/Professor . . ."** Josephine Ensign, "Disaster Tourism; All Right?," *Medical Margins* (blog), January 19, 2014, https://josephineensign.wordpress.com/2014/01/19/disaster-tourism-all-right/.

Witness: On Telling

30   **"Telling stories is as basic . . ."** Richard Kearney, *On Stories* (New York: Routledge, 2002), page 3.

30   **When trauma, illness, or injury occurs . . .**   This section is informed by Lars-Christer Hyden and Jens Brockmeier, eds., *Health, Illness and Culture: Broken Narratives* (New York: Routledge, 2008).

30   **Frank contends that there is a universal . . .** Arthur W. Frank, *The Wounded Storyteller: Body, Illness, and Ethics* (Chicago: The University of Chicago Press, 1995).

32   **The New Age, Joseph Campbell–like . . .** Joseph Campbell, Phil Cousineau, and Stuart L. Brown, *The Hero's Journey: The World of Joseph Campbell: Joseph Campbell on His Life and Work* (San Francisco: Harper & Row, 1990).

32-33   **"My father was a Presbyterian minister . . ."** Parts of this essay are adapted from Josephine Ensign, *Catching Homelessness: A Nurse's Story of Falling Through the Safety Net* (Berkeley: She Writes Press, 2016).

34   **Her "breaking the sequence" style of writing . . .** Virginia Woolf, "A Sketch from the Past," in *Moments of Being*, ed. Jeanne Schulkind (New York: A Harvest Book, 1985), page 72.

34   **Donnel B. Stern and "the unthought known" . . .** Donnel B. Stern, *Partners in Thought: Working with Unformulated Experience, Dissociation, and Enactment* (New York and London: Routledge, Taylor and Francis, 2009).

37   **"To tell one's life is to assume responsibility . . ."** Arthur W. Frank, *The Wounded Storyteller: Body, Illness, and Ethics* (Chicago: The University of Chicago Press, 1995), page xii.

37   **Witness is a relationship . . .** This is also informed by Arthur W. Frank, *Letting Stories Breathe: A Socio-Narratology* (Chicago: The University of Chicago Press, 2010).

38   **Feminist literary scholars Susan S. Lanser and Hélène Cixous . . .** Susan S. Lanser, "Toward a Feminist Narratology," *Style* 20, no. 3 (1986): 341–63; and Hélène Cixous, *White Ink: Interviews on Sex, Text, and Politics*, ed. Susan Sellers (New York: Columbia University Press, 2008).

38   **It requires more effort . . .** For more about broken narratives, see Arthur W. Frank, "Caring for the Dead: Broken Narratives of Internment," in Lars-Christer Hyden and Jens Brockmeier, eds., *Health, Illness and Culture: Broken Narratives* (New York: Routledge, 2008), 122–30. In this chapter, Frank describes broken narratives as "stories that resist telling; stories that the storyteller resists hearing himself or herself tell. The storyteller may self-consciously reflect on that resistance and make those reflections part of the story, or the storytelling may display resistance in gaps, inconsistencies, and other overt breaks in the narrative flow" (page 122).

Listen, Carefully

40   **"The fact that we are here . . ."** Audre Lorde, *The Cancer Journals* (San Francisco: Aunt Lute Books, 1997), page 22.

40   **Definition of slovenly: low, base . . .** *Oxford English Dictionary*, s.v. "slovenly," accessed October 10, 2015, http://www.oed.com.

41   **There's a** *Physician's Field Guide* **. . .** Frederic W. Platt and Geoffrey H.

Gordon, *Physician's Field Guide to the Difficult Patient Interview*, 2nd ed. (Philadelphia: Lippincott Williams and Wilkins, 2004).

42   *Listen carefully.* **To the pregnant pause . . .** My discussion of the uses of silence is informed by Cheryl Glenn and Krista Ratcliffe, *Silence and Listening as Rhetorical Arts* (Carbondale, IL: Southern Illinois University Press, 2011); Krista Ratcliffe, *Rhetorical Listening: Identification, Gender, Whiteness*, Studies in Rhetorics and Feminisms (Carbondale, IL: Southern Illinois University Press, 2005).

42   *Listen carefully.* **To the patient's illness narrative . . .** This section includes a critique of Rita Charon's narrative medicine close reading techniques as described in her book *Narrative Medicine: Honoring the Stories of Illness* (New York: Oxford University Press, 2006), and expanded upon in Rita Charon, Sayantani DasGupta, Nellie Hermann, Craig Irvine, Eric R. Marcus, Edgar Rivera Colón, Danielle Spencer, Maura Spiegel, *The Principles and Practice of Narrative Medicine* (New York: Oxford University Press, 2017).

Where the Homeless Go

This piece is written in the form of a *haibun*, which is autobiographical poetic prose accompanied by haiku. The piece is informed by the following sources: Bruce Ross, ed., *Journey to the Interior: American Versions of Haibun* (Boston: Tuttle Publishing, 1998); Matsuo Basho, *The Narrow Road to the Deep North and Other Travel Sketches,* trans. Nobuyuki Yuasa (New York: Penguin Books, 1966); and Howard Norman, "On the Poet's Trail," *National Geographic*, February 2008, http://ngm. nationalgeographic.com/2008/02/bashos-trail/howard-norman-text/1.

43   **"From this day forth . . ."** Basho, *Narrow Road*, page 72.

46   **"Each day is a journey . . ."** Matsuo Basho and David Landis Barnhill, *Basho's Journey: The Literary Prose of Matsuo Basho* (Ithaca, NY: State University of New York Press, 2005), page 49. The full quote: "For those who drift life away on a boat, for those who meet age leading a horse by the mouth, each day is a journey, the journey itself home."

Steps to Foot Care

This essay is based on an amalgam of real patients—their stories, their voices—and conversations between health science students and patients at a women's shelter in Seattle. The "Steps to Foot Care" instructions reproduced in this essay are the actual instructions on a printed form we give to our health science students when they provide foot care to people experiencing homelessness in Seattle-area homeless shelters. In health care, we check a person's pedal (foot) pulses on the inside of the ankle (posterior tibial) and on the top of the foot (dorsalis pedis) to assess the status of the circulatory system. In addition, we use a standardized piece of "fishing line" (microfilament) to touch various parts of a person's foot to assess for any neurological damage, especially that caused by uncontrolled diabetes.

47   **"It is appropriate that I sing . . ."** Nikki Giovanni, "The Song of the Feet," in *Quilting the Black-Eyed Pea* (New York: HarperCollins Publishers, 2002), page 110.

47-57   **"They think I gotta be stupid cause I talk all country-like."** I realize that my use of Southern dialect in this essay, which may appear to verge on what linguists term African American Vernacular English, can be viewed by some readers as inappropriate cultural appropriation. The main patient I had in mind while writing this essay was a white Southerner who grew up in poverty. As a Southerner, I can relate directly with this regional and class bias. An essay I found helpful while wrestling with this issue of cultural appropriation is Sarah Schulman's "White Writer," *The New Yorker*, October 21, 2016, http://www.newyorker.com/culture/cultural-comment/white-writer.

Footnotes

58   **"How many times these low feet . . ."** Emily Dickinson, "#187 How Many Times These Low Feet Staggered," in *Emily Dickinson: Selected Poems* (London: Phoenix Poetry, 2002), page 3.

58-60   **Footprints are witness to our beginnings . . .** For details on the history and science of dermatoglyphics, see Harold Cummins and Charles Midlo, *Finger Prints, Palms and Soles; An Introduction to Dermatoglyphics* (Philadelphia: Blakiston, 1943); Chris C. Plato, Ralph M. Garruto, and Blanka A. Schaumann, *Dermatoglyphics: Science in Transition* (New York: Wiley-Liss, 1991); Frankie L. Pack and Angela Dautartas, "Assessing the Correlation between Dermatoglyphics and Genetic Data in Worldwide Populations," *American Journal of Physical Anthropology* 150 (2013): 213–14; and Jamshed Mavalwala, ed., *Dermatoglyphics: An International Perspective, World Anthropology* (Stuttgart: De Gruyter Mouton, 2011).

58   **Not even identical twins . . .** Anahad O'Connor, "The Claim: Identical
Twins Have Identical Footprints," *The New York Times*, November 2,
2004, http://www.nytimes.com/2004/11/02/health/the-claim-identical-
twins-have-identical-fingerprints.html.

59   **Many Native American tribes consider feet sacred . . .** Sara Jean Green,
"Barefoot and . . . ," *Seattle Times: Pacific Northwest Magazine*, September
23, 2001, http://seattletimes.com/pacificnw/2001/0923/cover.html.

60   **Australian global health project called Happy Feet . . .**
"'Happy Feet' Biometrics Program Receives Gates Foundation Grant,"
Asian Scientist, December 12, 2011, http://www.asianscientist.
com/2011/12/tech/happy-feet-biometrics-infant-footprints-gates-
foundation-grand-challenges-explorations-grant-2011/.

Way Out; Way Home

61   **"Home? The edge of the alphabet . . ."** Janet Frame, *The Edge of the
Alphabet* (Christchurch, New Zealand: Pegasus Press, 1962), page 224.

61   **Ariadne was the daughter of . . .** For the myth of Ariadne, see Edward
McCrorie and Richard Martin, trans., *The Odyssey* (Baltimore: Johns
Hopkins University Press, 2004); Sophie Chiari, ed., *Renaissance Tales
of Desire: Hermaphroditus and Salmacis, Theseus and Ariadne, Ceyx and
Alcione* (Newcastle upon Tyne, UK: Cambridge Scholars Publishing,
2009); and Nina daVinci Nichols, *Ariadne's Lives* (Teaneck, NJ: Farleigh
Dickinson University Press, 1995).

65   **Blue is "something of an ecstatic accident . . ."** Maggie Nelson, *Bluets*
(Seattle: Wave Books, 2009), page 62.

65   **We love blue "because it draws us after it" . . .** Johann Wolfgang
von Goethe, *Theory of Colours*, trans. Charles Lock Eastlake
(London: John Murray, 1840), page 311, https://archive.org/details/
goethestheoryco01goetgoog. "But as we readily follow an agreeable object
that flies from us, so we love to contemplate blue, not because it advances
to us, but because it draws us after it."

66   **"Mirrors are filled with people . . ."** Eduardo Galeano, *Mirrors: Stories
of Almost Everyone*, trans. Mark Fried (New York: Nation Books, 2009),
page 1.

Past Forgiveness

This essay was informed by the work on the link between trauma, and especially childhood sexual abuse, and shame, including what has been termed "humiliated fury." Patricia Moran writes of this: "In other words, both the traumatic experience and the shame experience are imagistic, bodily based, and speechless, and so painful as to require banishment from consciousness." Patricia Moran, "Gunpowder Plots: Sexuality and Censorship in Woolf's Later Works," in *Virginia Woolf, Jean Rhys, and the Aesthetics of Trauma* (New York: Palgrave Macmillan, 2007), 67–89, page 81.

68   **"Forgetting is something that time alone . . ."** Simon Wiesenthal, *The Sunflower: On the Possibilities and Limits of Forgiveness* (New York: Schocken Books, 1997), pages 97–98.

68   **"There is simply too much injustice . . ."** Susan Sontag, *Regarding the Pain of Others* (New York: Picador, 2003), page 115.

68   **A young white supremacist shot . . .** Lizette Alvarez, "Charleston Families Hope Words Endure Past Shootings," *The New York Times*, June 24, 2015, http://www.nytimes.com/2015/06/25/us/charleston-families-hope-words-endure-past-shooting.html.

69   **In Judaism, forgiveness can only be . . .** Forgiveness within Judaism is discussed in Wiesenthal, *The Sunflower*.

69   **Forgiveness is also a peculiarly female thing . . .** Forgiveness as gendered is discussed in Sharon Lamb, "Women, Abuse, and Forgiveness: A Special Case," in *Before Forgiving: Cautionary Views of Forgiveness in Psychotherapy*, eds. Sharon Lamb and Jeffrie G. Murphy (London and New York: Oxford University Press, 2002), 155–71, as well as in Emily Yoffe, "The Debt," *Slate Magazine*, February 18, 2013, http://www.slate.com/articles/life/family/2013/02/abusive_parents_what_do_grown_children_owe_the_mothers_and_fathers_who_made.html.

69   **Robert Enright, a Catholic psychologist . . .** Robert D. Enright, *Forgiveness Is a Choice: A Step-by-Step Process for Resolving Anger and Restoring Hope* (Washington, DC: APA LifeTools, 2001).

69   **An International Forgiveness Day . . .** World Wide Forgiveness Alliance, accessed September 1, 2017, http://www.forgivenessalliance.org/forgiveness-day.php.

70   **Thirty-three-item online forgiveness quiz . . .** This 33-item forgiveness quiz was based on psychology professor Warren H. Jones's individual differences research; I took the quiz on November 5, 2015, at http://

www.thepowerofforgiveness.com/quiz/ (site now discontinued).

70   **"To err is human; to forgive, divine."** Alexander Pope, "An Essay on
Criticism, Written in the Year 1709," in *Pope, Alexander: The Works
(1736)* (University of Pennsylvania Department of Linguistics), vol.
1, with explanatory notes and additions never before printed, http://
languagelog.ldc.upenn.edu/myl/ldc/ling001/pope_crit.htm.

70   **I question our society's insistence on forgiveness . . .** Vidhya I.
Kamat, Warren H. Jones, and Kathleen L. Row, "Assessing Forgiveness
as a Dimension of Personality," *Individual Differences Research* 4, no. 5
(December 2006): 322–30.

70   **Wallace Stegner's "native home of hope" . . .** Wallace Stegner, *The
Sound of Mountain Water* (New York: Dutton, 1980), page 38.

73   **The scar is still there . . .**   Donnel B. Stern, *Partners in Thought:
Working with Unformulated Experience, Dissociation, and Enactment*
(London and New York: Routledge, 2009).

The Body Remembers

74   **"Let us turn our pain to power . . ."** Eve Ensler, *In the Body of the World*
(New York: Metropolitan Books, 2013), page 216.

74   **"What kind of beast would turn its life . . ."** Adrienne Rich, *The Dream
of a Common Language* (New York: W. W. Norton and Company, 2013),
page 28.

74   **"It was an old theme even for me . . ."** Rich, *Dream of a Common
Language*, page 19.

75   **The research technique of discourse analysis . . .** Ruth Wodak and
Michael Meyer, eds., *Methods of Critical Discourse Analysis* (London: Sage
Publications, 2002).

75   **Listening for evidence of Foucault's "counter-memories" . . .**
Michel Foucault, *Language, Counter-Memory, Practice: Selected Essays and
Interviews*, ed. Donald F. Bouchard (Ithaca, NY: Cornell University Press,
1977); Jose Medina, "Toward a Foucaultian Epistemology of Resistance:
Counter-Memory, Epistemic Friction, and Guerrilla Pluralism," *Foucault
Studies* 12 (October 2011): 9–35.

76   **The conference workshop I refer to . . .** Elizabeth K. Hopper, Ellen L.
Bassuk, and Jeffrey Olivet, "Shelter from the Storm: Trauma-Informed
Care in Homelessness Services Settings," *The Open Health Services and*

Policy Journal 3 (2010): 80–100.

77   **An illness that casts a shadow . . .** Arthur W. Frank, "Tricksters
      and Truth Tellers: Narrating Illness in an Age of Authenticity and
      Appropriation," *Literature and Medicine* 28, no. 2 (Fall 2009): 185–99.

77   **"All trauma is preverbal . . ."** Bessel van der Kolk, *The Body Keeps
      the Score: Brain, Mind, and Body in the Healing of Trauma* (New York:
      Penguin Books, 2014), page 43.

77   **"Almost every brain-imaging study . . ."** Van der Kolk, *Body Keeps the
      Score,* page 249.

78   **"In other words trauma makes . . ."** Van der Kolk, *Body Keeps the Score,*
      page 249.

78   **"And if the text stands for . . ."** Laurence J. Kirmayer, "The Body's
      Insistence on Meaning: Metaphor as Presentation and Representation
      in Illness Experience," *Medical Anthropology Quarterly* 6, no. 4 (1992):
      323–46, pages 324–25.

78-79 **Maddy Coy, a UK-based researcher . . .** Maddy Coy, "This Body Which
      Is Not Mine: The Notion of the Habit Body, Prostitution and (Dis)
      embodiment," *Feminist Theory* 10, no. 1 (2009): 61–75.

79   **"Untenable and destructive" expectations . . . and "People who
      have been effective . . ."** Laura van Dernoot Lipsky with Connie Burk,
      *Trauma Stewardship: An Everyday Guide to Caring for Self While Caring
      for Others* (San Francisco: Berrett-Koehler Publishers, 2009), page 159.

79   **Eve Ensler and her personal work . . .** Ensler, *In the Body.*

79   **Language does appear to be important . . .** For resources about the
      role of language in development of a healthy sense of self, see A. D.
      Peterkin and A. A. Prettyman, "Finding a Voice: Revisiting the History of
      Therapeutic Writing," *Medical Humanities* 35 (2009): 80–88; and James
      W. Pennebaker, *Opening Up: The Healing Power of Expressing Emotions*
      (The Guilford Press: London, 1997).

79-80 **In his influential article "Against Narrativity" . . .** Galen Strawson,
      "Against Narrativity," *Ratio* 17, no. 4 (December 4, 2004): 428–52.

80   **"Western, middle-class, liberal and neoliberal . . ."** Angela Woods,
      "The Limits of Narrative: Provocations for the Medical Humanities,"
      Medical Humanities 37 (2011): 73–78, page 76. Also informed by Angela
      Woods, "Beyond the Wounded Storyteller: Rethinking Narrativity,
      Illness and Embodied Self-Experience," in *Health, Illness and Disease:*

Philosophical Essays, eds. Havi Carel and Rachel Cooper (Newcastle, UK: Acumen, 2012), 113–28.

80   **Contrary to the common cheery . . .** Van der Kolk, *Body Keeps the Score*, page 196.

80   **As Arthur Frank reminds us, telling . . .** Arthur W. Frank, *The Wounded Storyteller: Body, Illness, and Ethics* (Chicago: The University of Chicago Press, 1995).

80-81   **"The dilemma writers face is . . ."** Louise DeSalvo, *Writing as a Way of Healing: How Telling Our Stories Transforms Our Lives* (Boston: Beacon Press, 1999), page 163.

81   **"Telling one's own story is good . . ."** Arthur W. Frank, "Tricksters and Truth Tellers: Narrating Illness in an Age of Authenticity and Appropriation," *Literature and Medicine* 28, no. 2 (Fall 2009): 185–99, page 196.

81   **An intriguing example of a stolen story . . .** Anna Thiemann, "Reversing the Commodification of Life? Rebecca Skloot's Narrative Science Writing," in *The Writing Cure: Literature and Medicine in Context*, eds. Alexandra Lembert-Heidenreich and Jarmila Mildorf (Berlin: Lit Verlag Dr. W. Hopf., 2013), 191–210.

81   **"The three most important things . . ."** Vanessa Northington Gamble, "Subcutaneous Scars," *Health Affairs* 19, no. 1 (February 2000): 164–69, page 169.

Endurance Test

83   **"This fevered exploration of both . . ."** "Katherine Boo: By the Book," *The New York Times Sunday Book Review*, February 7, 2013, http://www.nytimes.com/2013/02/10/books/review/katherine-boo-by-the-book.html.

83-92   **An explosion of research on resilience . . .** For more critiques of resilience, post-traumatic stress disorder (PTSD), and community resilience, see Paul Farmer, "On Suffering and Structural Violence: A View from Below," in *Violence in War and Peace*, eds. Nancy Scheper-Hughes and Philippe Bourgois (New York: Blackwell Publishing, 2004), 281–89; Pierre Bourdieu, *In Other Words: Essays Towards a Reflexive Sociology* (Stanford, CA: Stanford University Press, 1990); Jaimie Hicks Masterson, Walter Gillis Peacock, Shannon S. Van Zandt, Himanshu

Grover, Lori Field Schwarz, and John T. Cooper Jr., *Planning for Community Resilience: A Handbook for Reducing Vulnerability to Disasters* (Washington, DC: Island Press, 2014); Matthew J. Friedman, Terence M. Keane, and Patricia A. Resick, eds., *Handbook of PTSD: Science and Practice*, 2nd ed. (New York: The Guilford Press, 2014); and Brad Evans and Julian Reid, *Resilient Life: The Art of Living Dangerously* (Cambridge, UK: Polity Press, 2014).

83   **American Psychological Association definition of** *resilience . . .* "The Road to Resilience," American Psychological Association, Psychology Help Center, accessed September 1, 2017, http://www.apa.org/helpcenter/road-resilience.aspx.

84   **Most research on resilience has focused . . .** Martha Kent, Mary C. Davies, and John W. Reich, eds., *The Resilience Handbook: Approaches to Stress and Trauma* (New York: Routledge, 2014).

84   **Resilience-building interventions include . . .** Martha Kent and Mary C. Davies, "Resilience Training for Action and Agency to Stress and Trauma: Becoming the Hero of Your Life," in *The Resilience Handbook*, eds. Kent, Davies, and Reich, 227–44.

84   **Therapies aimed at increasing social support . . .** Mary H. Burleson and Mary C. Davis, "Social Touch and Resilience," in *The Resilience Handbook*, eds. Kent, Davies, and Reich, 131–43.

84   **"The world breaks everyone . . ."** Ernest Hemingway, *A Farewell to Arms* (New York: Charles Scribner's Sons, 1957), page 249.

85   **"The capacity to suffer is, clearly . . ."** Paul Farmer, "On Suffering and Structural Violence: A View from Below," in *Violence in War and Peace*, eds. Scheper-Hughes and Bourgois, 281–89, page 288.

85   **"And I mean by endure withstand . . ."** Arthur Kleinman, "The Art of Medicine: How We Endure," *The Lancet* 383 (January 11, 2014): 119–20, page 119.

88   **A Katrina National Memorial Park . . .** Katrina National Memorial Park, Katrina National Memorial Foundation, http://www.knmfno.org/the-project/.

89   **This Katrina memorial was created by "Dr. Frank Minyard . . ."** For information on and interviews with Dr. Frank Minyard, see PBS Frontline's video *Post Mortem: Death Investigation in America* (Boston: WGBH Educational Foundation, 2011), http://www.pbs.org/wgbh/

pages/frontline/post-mortem/.

89   **The permanent exhibit** *Living with Hurricanes* . . . The exhibit was
        Living With Hurricanes: Katrina and Beyond, in the Lousiana State
        Museum, The Presbytére, http://louisianastatemuseum.org/museums/
        the-presbytere/.

89   *Message of Remembrances (2010)*, **by Mitchell Gaudet** . . . For
        information on the artist Mitchell Gaudet, see Doug MacCash, "'Katrina
        X' Exhibit in Arabi Recalls 2005 With Grace and Grit," *The Times-
        Picayune* (New Orleans), August 20, 2015, http://www.nola.com/arts/
        index.ssf/2015/08/studio_inferno_mitchell_gaudet.html.

90   **An iconic image by Eudora Welty** . . . Eudora Welty, "Home with
        Bottle-Trees, Simpson County," The Mississippi Writers Page, The
        University of Mississippi, accessed September 1, 2017, http://mwp.
        olemiss.edu//dir/welty_eudora/bottle_trees.html.

90   **The folk belief is that** . . . Jeff Kid, "Blue-Bottle Trees: A Throwback
        to Gullah Tradition," *The Beaufort Gazette*, December 11, 2009, http://
        www.lowcountrynewspapers.net/archive/node/145052.

91   **But one section of the Katrina exhibit** . . . Elizabeth Mullener, "After
        Hurricane Katrina Struck, Elton Mabry Used Writing as a Way to
        Survive the Storm," *The Times-Picayune* (New Orleans), August 23, 2008,
        http://blog.nola.com/elizabethmullener/2008/08/jennifer_zdon_the_
        timespicayun.html.

92   **Tommy Elton Mabry died of** . . . Elizabeth Mullener, "Hurricaine
        Katrina Survivor and Chronicler Tommy Mabry Dies at 58," *The Times-
        Picayune* (New Orleans), February 1, 2013, http://www.nola.com/
        katrina/index.ssf/2013/02/hurricane_katrina_survivor_tom.html.

92   **"Means repair but it also means transformation . . ."** Veena Das and
        Arthur Kleinman, "Introduction," in *Remaking a World: Violence, Social
        Suffering, and Recovery*, eds. Veena Das, Arthur Kleinman, Margaret
        Lock, Mamphela Ramphele, and Pamela Reynolds (Berkeley: University
        of California Press, 2001), 1–30, page 23.

An Over-Examined Life

93   **"Coming home at last . . ."** Matsuo Basho, *The Narrow Road to the
        Deep North and Other Travel Sketches,* trans. Nobuyuki Yuasa (New York:
        Penguin Books, 1966), page 77.

95   **The word** *journal* **derives from . . .**   *Oxford English Dictionary*, s.v. "journal" and "diary," accessed December 15, 2015, http://www.oed.com.

95   **The Journalate tagline "Empty your head. Privately."** Journalate home page, https://journalate.com/.

96   **Earliest examples of journals? Augustine's** *Confessions* **. . .** Saint Augustine, *The Confessions of Saint Augustine*, trans. E. B. Pusey (401; Project Gutenberg, 2002), E-book #3296, https://www.gutenberg.org/files/3296/3296-h/3296-h.htm.

96   **"My records are little more than . . ."** Basho, *Narrow Road,* page 74.

97   **"These rough notes and our dead bodies . . ."** Robert Falcon Scott, "Scott's Last Expedition," from *The Journals of Captain R. F. Scott* (1913), published online at the University of Cambridge, Scott Polar Research Institute, http://www.spri.cam.ac.uk/museum/diaries/scottslastexpedition/, "Message to the Public, March 29, 1912."

97   **Both Thomas Jefferson and Benjamin Franklin . . .**   Peter Stallybrass, "Benjamin Franklin: Printed Corrections and Erasable Writing," *Proceedings of the American Philosophical Society* 150, no. 4 (December 2006): 553–67.

97   **The famous female-only "rest cure". . .** Charlotte Perkins Gilman, *The Yellow Wallpaper* (Boston: Small and Maynard, 1899).

98   **"Swan's day-upon-day sluice . . ."**   Ivan Doig, *Winter Brothers: A Season at the Edge of America* (New York: Harcourt Brace Jovanovich, 1980), 65–66, page 65.

98   **The decade-long, million-word diary . . .** Samuel Pepys, *The Diary of Samuel Pepys* (1893; Project Gutenberg, 2003), E-book 4200, http://www.gutenberg.org/ebooks/4200.

99   **"We commonly do not remember . . ."** Henry Thoreau, *Walden and Civil Disobedience* (New York: Penguin Books, 1983), page 45.

99   **"Between 1837 and 1861, Thoreau . . ."** Andrea Wulf, "A Man for All Seasons," *The New York Times Sunday Book Review*, April 19, 2013, http://www.nytimes.com/2013/04/21/books/review/a-man-for-all-seasons.html.

100   **"And when is there time to remember . . ."** Tillie Olsen, "I Stand Here Ironing," in *Tell Me a Riddle* (New York: Dell Publishing, 1994), page XX; see also Tillie Olsen, *Silences* (New York: Delacorte Press/Seymour

Lawrence, 1978).

100   **"Somedays [sic], if bitterness were a whetstone . . ."** Audre Lorde, *The Cancer Journals* (San Francisco: Aunt Lute Books, 1997), page 13.

100   **She gave a speech at Amherst College . . .** Audre Lorde, "Age, Race, Class, and Sex: Women Redefining Difference," in *Sister Outsider: Essays and Speeches* (Berkeley: Crossing Press, 2007), quotations from page 116.

101   **"When I opened my mother's journals . . ."** Terry Tempest Williams, *When Women Were Birds: Fifty-Four Variations on Voice* (New York: Farrar, Straus and Giroux, 2012), page 22.

103   **C. S. Lewis's admonition that journal writing . . .** C. S. Lewis, *A Grief Observed* (New York: HarperCollins, 2009).

104   **"Keepers of private notebooks are . . ."** Joan Didion, "On Keeping a Notebook," in *Slouching Towards Bethlehem* (New York: Farrar, Straus and Giroux, 2008), 131–41, pages 132–33.

104   **"From the beginning, I knew . . ."** Sarah Manguso, *Ongoingness: The End of a Diary* (Minneapolis, MN: Graywolf Press, 2015), page 4.

104   **"He is the most acute of observers . . ."** Joyce Carol Oates, "Inspiration and Obsession in Life and Literature," *The New York Review of Books*, August 13, 2015, http://www.nybooks.com/articles/2015/08/13/inspiration-and-obsession-life-and-literature/.

104-5   **"Is the keeping of a journal . . ."** Joyce Carol Oates, "Introduction," in *The Journal of Joyce Carol Oates, 1973–1982*, ed. Greg Johnson (New York: HarperCollins, 2007), i–xiv, page xii.

105   **Journal writing is a lifeline . . .** For more about the role of narration in the development of self-identity, see Michael Bamberg, "Who Am I? Narration and Its Contribution to Self and Identity," *Theory & Psychology* 21, no. 1 (2011): 3–24; Deborah Schiffrin, Anna De Fina, and Anastasia Nylund, *Telling Stories: Language, Narrative, and Social Life*, Georgetown University Round Table on Languages and Linguistics Series (Washington, DC: Georgetown University Press, 2010); Anthony Giddens, *Modernity and Self-Identity: Self and Society in the Late Modern Age* (Redwood City, CA: Stanford University Press, 1991); Cheryl Mattingly, "Moral Selves and Moral Scenes: Narrative Experiments in Everyday Life," *Ethnos* 78, no. 3 (2013): 301–27; and Cheryl Mattingly, *Healing Dramas and Narrative Plots: The Narrative Structure of Experience* (Cambridge, UK: Cambridge University Press, 1998).

105   **The long line of people imprisoned . . .** For general information on journal writing, see Curtis W. Casewit, *The Diary: A Complete Guide to Journal Writing* (Allen, TX: Argus Communications, 1982); Christina Baldwin, *Life's Companion: Journal Writing as a Spiritual Quest* (New York: Bantam Books, 1991); Kate Thompson, *Therapeutic Journal Writing: An Introduction for Professionals* (London: Jessica Kingsley Publishers, 2011); and Sheila Bender, *Keeping a Journal You Love* (Cincinnati, OH: Walking Stick Press, 2001).

106   **My journals as primary source material . . .** Josephine Ensign, *Catching Homelessness: A Nurse's Story of Falling Through the Safety Net* (Berkeley: She Writes Press, 2016).

106   **"I note however that this diary . . ."** Virginia Woolf, *A Writer's Diary: Being Extracts from the Diary of Virginia Woolf*, ed. Leonard Woolf (London: The Hogarth Press, 1953), page 7.

106   **"I'm interested in depression . . ."** Virginia Woolf, quoted in Louise DeSalvo, *Virginia Woolf: The Impact of Childhood Sexual Abuse on Her Life and Work* (Boston: Beacon Press, 1989), page 99.

107   **Virginia Woolf spoke with her sister . . .** Virginia Woolf, "A Sketch from the Past," in *Moments of Being*, ed. Jeanne Schulkind, (New York: A Harvest Book, 1985).

107   **People have tried to use as evidence . . .** In his introduction to *A Passionate Apprentice: The Early Journals of Virginia Woolf* (London: The Hogarth Press, 1990), editor Mitchell A. Leaska goes to great lengths to question whether sexual abuse even happened, stating this: "The Duckworth brothers [Virginia's older half-brothers], guilty as they might have been of sexual interference, very probably become the despised objects on to which she could attach the deeply disturbing fantasy she herself harboured (sic) for her father" (page xxxv).

108   **"We are paranoid about privacy . . ."** Christina Baldwin, *One to One: Self-Understanding Through Journal Writing* (New York: M. Evans and Company, 1991), page 43.

108   **"Organ donation provides an apt analogy . . ."** Casey N. Cep, "Books and Bodies: On Organs and Literary Estates," *The Daily* (blog), *The Paris Review*, August 22, 2012, http://www.theparisreview.org/ blog/2012/08/22/books-and-bodies-on-organs-and-literary-estates/.

108   **There are the famous examples . . .** Nicolette Jones, "Fame Beyond the

Grave," *The Telegraph*, July 3, 2009, http://www.telegraph.co.uk/culture/books/bookreviews/5720775/Fame-beyond-the-grave.html.

108   **"Would you destroy all my papers."** Virginia Woolf, quoted in DeSalvo, *Virginia Woolf: The Impact of Childhood Sexual Abuse*, page 133.

108-9   **"Burned manuscripts are a death . . ."** Jones, "Fame Beyond the Grave," http://www.telegraph.co.uk/culture/books/bookreviews/5720775/Fame-beyond-the-grave.html.

109   **"Two more notebooks survived . . ."** Frances McCullough, ed., and Ted Hughes, consulting ed., *The Journals of Sylvia Plath* (New York: The Dial Press, 1982), page xiii.

109   **He reports that Plath was rereading . . .** This is informed by Ted Hughes's article "Sylvia Plath and Her Journals," *Grand Street* 1 (1982): 86–99.

109   **She was working on her memoir . . .** Sylvia Plath, *The Bell Jar* (New York: Harper Collins, 2006).

109   **In the seemingly never-ending tragedy . . .** Margaret Drabble, "Son of Poets Sylvia Plath and Ted Hughes Kills Himself," *The Guardian,* March 23, 2009, http://www.theguardian.com/books/2009/mar/23/sylvia-plath-son-kills-himself.

110   **"He provided this service to . . ."** Heidi Julavits, "Mostly True: Two Writers and One Artist Reflect on the Slipperiest of All Literary Forms—Their Own Diaries," *The New York Times Style Magazine*, February 13, 2015, http://www.nytimes.com/2015/02/13/t-magazine/sarah-manguso-amalia-ulman-heidi-julavits-diary.html.

110   **The multiple positive health effects of writing . . .** James W. Pennebaker, "Writing, Social Processes, and Psychotherapy," in *The Writing Cure: How Expressive Writing Promotes Health and Emotional Well-Being*, eds. Stephen J. Lepore and Joshua M. Smyth (Washington, DC: American Psychological Association, 2002), 281–291.

111   **Perhaps a different sort of overexamined life . . .** Kit Boss, "A Life, Single Spaced—Can A 36Million-Word Diary Capture a Man?—The Diarist of Dayton for 22 Years, Five Minutes at a Time, Rev. Robert Shields Transforms The Ordinary Into Something Else," *The Seattle Times*, May 15, 1994, http://community.seattletimes.nwsource.com/archive/?date=19940515&slug=1910502.

111   **When Shields died, in 2007 . . .** Douglas Martin, "Robert Shields,

Wordy Diarist, Dies at 89," *The New York Times*, October 29, 2007.

111   **As Andrea Wulf reports . . .** Wulf, "A Man for All Seasons," http://www.
nytimes.com/2013/04/21/books/review/a-man-for-all-seasons.html.

112   **"I shall not again desert . . ."** Virginia Woolf, *A Passionate Apprentice:
The Early Journals of Virginia Woolf*, ed. Mitchell A. Leaska (London: The
Hogarth Press, 1990), page 71.

114   **"To so many black films . . ."** Woolf, *A Writer's Diary*, page 7.

Lab Notebook

116   **"Tell me, what is it you plan to do . . ."** Mary Oliver, *New and Collected
Poems: Volume One* (Boston: Beacon Press, 1992), page 94.

117   **According to Robert E. Ornstein . . .** Robert E. Ornstein, *The Psychology
of Consciousness* (New York: Harcourt Brace Jovanovich, 1977), pages
16–39.

118   **Afterword of** *A Grief Observed . . .*   Chad Walsh, "Afterword," in C. S.
Lewis's *A Grief Observed* (New York: Bantam Books, 1976), 93–150.

118   **Continuing to read** *The Psychology . . .* Ornstein, *The Psychology of
Consciousness*, 155.

118   **"Ordinary language is structured to follow . . ."** Arthur J. Deikman,
"Deautomatization and the Mystic Experience," *Psychiatry* 29, no. 4
(1966), 324–38, page 338.

118-19 **In** *The Pilgrim's Regress* **I note . . .** C. S. Lewis, *The Pilgrim's Regress: An
Allegorical Apology for Christianity, Reason and Romanticism* (London:
Geoffrey Bles, 1943).

119   **In my private reading professor Gilbert . . .** Gilbert Meilaender, *The
Taste for the Other: The Social and Ethical Thought of C. S. Lewis* (Grand
Rapids, MI: William B. Eerdmans, 1978).

119   **Lewis's fantasy book** *Till We . . .* C. S. Lewis, *Till We Have Faces*
(London: Geoffrey Bes, 1956).

120   **Lewis claims that myth does not . . .** Corbin Scott Carnell, *Bright
Shadow of Reality: C. S. Lewis and the Feeling Intellect* (Grand Rapids, MI:
William B. Eerdmans, 1974), 106.

121   **Carl Sagan, in** *The Dragons . . .* Carl Sagan, *The Dragons of Eden:
Speculations on the Evolution of Human Intelligence* (New York: Random
House, 1977).

121   **In his autobiography,** *Surprised by Joy . . .* C. S. Lewis, *Surprised by Joy:*

The Shape of My Early Life (New York: Harcourt, Brace & Company, 1955); see especially chapter 1, "The First Years," pages 3–21.

122   **Carl Sagan writes of . . . and Sagan points out that . . .** Sagan, *Dragons of Eden*, 127–28.

122   **"You may add that in the hive . . ."** Lewis, *Surprised by Joy*, pages 8–9.

123   **From Robert S. Ellwood Jr.'s book . . .** Robert S. Ellwood Jr., *Religious and Spiritual Groups in Modern America* (Englewood Cliffs, NJ: Prentice-Hall, Inc.); see especially cha1, "In Quest of New Religions," pages 1–41, and cha2, "The History of An Alternative Reality in the West," pages 42–87.

123   **Lewis claims that . . . and Lewis contends that . . .** C. S. Lewis, *The Weight of Glory* (New York: Macmillan, 1949).

124   **While reading** *The Psychology of Consciousness* . . . Ornstein, *The Psychology of Consciousness*, especially cha11, "An Extended Concept of Human Consciousness," pages 214–33.

124   **"I can never again believe . . ."** C. S. Lewis, *A Grief Observed* (New York: Bantam Books, 1976), page 6.

124-25 **C. S. Lewis biographers surmise that . . .** A. N. Wilson, *C. S. Lewis: A Biography* (New York: W. W. Norton, 1990).

125   **"The feelings, acts and experiences . . ."** William James, *The Varieties of Religious Experience: A Study in Human Nature* (New York: Random House, 1902), pages 31–2.

125   **"The victory of vivisection marks . . ."** C. S. Lewis, *God in the Dock: Essays on Theology and Ethics* (Grand Rapids, MI: William B. Eerdmans, 1970), 224–228, page 228.

126-27 **"'Who—or what—am I?' . . ."** Arthur J. Deikman, "The Missing Center," in *Alternate States of Consciousness*, ed. E. Zinberg (New York: The Free Press, 1977), 230–241, page 241.

127   **Things I gleaned from reading Corbin . . .** Carnell, *Bright Shadow of Reality*.

127   **William James contends that personal . . .** James, *Varieties of Religious Experience*, see especially "Lectures XVI and XVII: Mysticism," pages 378–9.

128   **"If love is only lust . . ."** Carnell, *Bright Shadow of Reality,* page 137.

128-29 **Lewis included in** *The Four Loves* . . . C. S. Lewis, *The Four Loves* (San Diego, CA: Harcourt Brace Jovanovich, 1960), 105–11.

Medical Maze

130   **"Who's turned us around like this . . ."** Rainer Maria Rilke, *Duino Elegies and the Sonnets to Orpeus*, trans. A. Poulin Jr. (Boston: Houghton Mifflin Company, 2005), page 59.

130   **I work in the world's largest . . .** See "Work Smarter, Not Larger," NBJJ Architecture Company, accessed September 1, 2017, http://www.nbbj.com/work/university-of-washington-health-sciences-center-t-wing-teaching-space/.

130   **More than thirty Walmart Supercenters . . .** Walmart Supercenters "are around 182,000 square feet," according to Walmart's webpage "Our Business," accessed September 1, 2017, http://corporate.walmart.com/our-story/our-business.

131   **"Spinach green" is what Harry Sherman . . .** David Pantalony, "The Colour of Medicine," *Canadian Medical Association Journal* 181, no. 6–7 (September 15, 2009): 402–3.

131   **"The convalescent needs the positive colors . . ."** William O. Ludlow, "Color in the Modern Hospital," *The Modern Hospital* 16, no. 6, (June 1921): 511–13, page 511.

131   **Color-coding of medical center hallways . . .** Barbara J. Huelat, *Wayfinding: Design for Understanding*, A Position Paper for the Center for Health Design's Environmental Standards Council (Concord, CA: The Center for Health Design), October 2007, http://www.healthdesign.org/chd/research/wayfinding-design-understanding.

131   **"In the kingdom of the well . . ."** Susan Sontag, *Illness as Metaphor* (New York: Farrar, Straus and Giroux, 1978), page 3.

132   **A prime example of brutalism . . .**   "Brutalism," Washington State Department of Archaeology and Historic Preservation, accessed September 1, 2017, http://www.dahp.wa.gov/styles/brutalism.

133   **Langlie laid a ceremonial cornerstone . . .** Cassandra Tate, "University of Washington Health Sciences Building Is Dedicated on October 9, 1949," HistoryLink.org, Essay 10177 (December 10, 2012), http://www.historylink.org/index.cfm?DisplayPage=output.cfm&file_id=10177.

133   **Cornerstone, foundation stone, quoin stone . . .** For more about cornerstones and quoin stones, see William E. Jarvis, *Time Capsules: A Cultural History* (Jefferson, NC: McFarland & Company, 2003); James George Frazer, *The Golden Bough* (Oxford and New York: Oxford

University Press, 1998), 162–63; and Toni Maraini, *Sealed in Stone*, trans. A. K. Bierman (San Francisco: City Lights Books, 2002).

133   **The modern hospital traces its roots . . .** For more on the history of hospitals, see Guenter B. Risse, *Mending Bodies, Saving Souls: A History of Hospitals* (New York: Oxford University Press, 1999).

134   **"The walls palpitate to the rhythm . . ."** Richard Selzer, "Down from Troy, Part 1," in *The Exact Location of the Soul: New and Selected Essays* (New York: Picador, 2001), 23–42, page 33.

135-36   **I thought of Kafka's** *Metamorphosis* . . . Franz Kafka, *Metamorphosis*, trans. David Wyllie (2002; Project Gutenberg, 2005) E-book #5200, http://www.gutenberg.org/files/5200/5200-h/5200-h.htm.

136   **Malaise, from the Old French** *mal* . . . *Oxford English Dictionary*, s.v. "malaise," accessed June 21, 2015, http://www.oed.com.

Degree of Latitude

139   **"There is wild in us yet . . ."** Brian Doyle, *The Sun*, March 2016, page 23.

139   **This is a test of your mental state . . .** The mental test items presented at the beginning of this essay are based on the Mini-Mental State Examination (MMSE), a common neurocognitive test used by health professionals to screen patients for dementia or other cognitive deficits. The questions and instructions in parentheses are ones I created. The MMSE is available online from the University of Massachusetts Lowell, accessed September 1, 2017, https://www.uml.edu/docs/Mini Mental State Exam_tcm18-169319.pdf.

141   **We develop cognitive maps—mental maps . . .** For more on neurocognitive direction-finding, see Hugo J. Spiers and Eleanor A. Maguire, "Thoughts, Behaviour, and Brain Dynamics during Navigation in the Real World," *NeuroImage* 33 (April 11, 2006): 1826–40; Lawrence K. Altman, "Nobel Prize in Medicine Is Awarded to Three Who Discovered Brain's 'Inner GPS,'" *The New York Times*, October 6, 2014, http://www.nytimes.com/2014/10/07/science/nobel-prize-medicine.html.

143   **Entering a new and dramatic territory . . .** Christopher J. Preston, *Grounding Knowledge: Environmental Philosophy, Epistemology, and Place* (Athens: University of Georgia Press, 2003).

144   **Past events of great importance . . .** Keith H. Basso, *Wisdom Sits in*

Places: Landscape and Language among the Western Apache (Albuquerque: The University of New Mexico Press, 1996).

Epilogue

145   **William James's** *The Varieties of . . .* William James, *The Varieties of Religious Experience: A Study in Human Nature* (New York: Random House, 1902)

146   **Susan Sontag's book** *Illness as Metaphor . . .* Susan Sontag, *Illness as Metaphor* (New York: Farrar, Straus and Giroux, 1978).

146   **My medical memoir,** *Catching Homelessness . . .* Josephine Ensign, *Catching Homelessness: A Nurse's Story of Falling Through the Safety Net* (Berkeley: She Writes Press, 2016).

147   **"What I'm ultimately interested in is teaching people . . ."** Wise words from Sayantani DasGupta, "Narrative Medicine, Narrative Humility: Listening to the Streams of Stories," *Creative Nonfiction* (Summer 2014), 6–7, page 7.

Index to Authors and Artists Cited

About the Author

Josephine Ensign is professor of nursing at the University of Washington (UW) in Seattle, where she teaches health policy, population health, and health humanities. She is adjunct professor in the UW School of Arts and Sciences, Department of Gender, Women and Sexuality Studies, as well as affiliate faculty at the UW Simpson Center for the Humanities. She received her bachelor's degree (biology and religion) from Oberlin College, her master's degree in primary care nursing from the Medical College of Virginia, and her doctorate in public health from Johns Hopkins University. Ensign has worked as a family nurse practitioner and health services researcher for the past three decades, focusing on primary health care for homeless adolescents and adults in the United States, as well as in Thailand, Venezuela, and New Zealand. She is the author of numerous academic and narrative medicine journal articles, as well as the narrative policy book *Catching Homelessness: A Nurse's Story of Falling Through the Safety Net*, which was named the *American Journal of Nursing* 2017 Book of the Year for Creative Works. Ensign writes a blog, *Medical Margins*, on health humanities, policy, and nursing.